TABLE OF CONTENTS

James C. Reynolds, M.D.

PATHOPHYSIOLOGY AND CLINICAL ASPECTS OF PEPTIC ULCER DISEASE

THERAPY OF PEPTIC ULCER DISEASE

Arthur J. Atkinson, Jr., M.D.
and Robert M. Craig, M.D.

LIST OF ILLUSTRATIONS

Peptic acid diseases include a constellation of disorders ranging from irritation of the stomach or the esophagus, on the one hand, to frank ulceration most commonly seen in the duodenum or stomach. Given the caustic nature of gastric contents, it is not surprising that ulceration can occur. One might even expect the incidence of such disorders to be far higher than it is. Be that as it may, the fact remains that these diseases have been responsible for enormous suffering, and catastrophic sequelae, including perforation and severe hemorrhage, which have been associated with significant mortality.

Until the discovery of H_2-receptor antagonists by Sir James Black, working at SmithKline and French Laboratories in Welwyn, England, the management of patients with peptic acid disease was largely palliative and not particularly effective. Dietary regulation was a prominent feature of most therapeutic regimens. Diets often were limited to bland foods, and patients were instructed to eat multiple meals per day for periods of months, if not years. Other major lifestyle changes were recommended that were designed to reduce stress, in the hope that this would lower the frequency of recurrence. If these measures failed, vagotomy and pyloroplasty were used to reduce acid secretion and accelerate gastric emptying. Subtotal gastrectomy was an approach of last resort for patients with severe and intractable disease. These surgical procedures were accompanied by their own attendant morbidity and mortality.

This bleak situation changed dramatically with the release of cimetidine, an H_2-receptor antagonist. The discovery of cimeditine is one of the great triumphs of modern pharmacology and medicine. Much of the credit goes to Sir James Black who already had been responsible for the development of propranolol, a ß-adrenergic receptor antagonist. By analogy to the α- and ß-adrenergic receptor subtypes, each of which could be blocked selectively by appropriate drugs, he thought that there might be multiple classes of histamine receptor. A variety of antihistaminic compounds had been synthesized. Many of these compounds were centrally active, and they blocked the effects of histamine on blood pressure. These compounds did not, however, block the effect of histamine as a stimulant of gastric acid secretion. The hypothesis developed was that there were two classes of histamine receptor, called H_1 and H_2. Black's accomplishment was to validate this hypothesis, to develop *in vitro* assays that would allow him to distinguish between effects mediated at H_1 and H_2 receptors, and ultimately to identify compounds that would selectively block H_2 receptors and reduce gastric acid secretion without blocking H_1 receptors. After investigating the properties of over 200 compounds, a lead compound, $N\alpha$-guanylhistamine, was discovered in 1968. Success ultimately came in 1974 with a cyano derivative called cyanoguanidine, or cimetidine, ultimately marketed under the name Tagamet®.

In addition to H_2-receptor antagonists, it is now possible to treat and cure peptic ulcer disease with a variety of agents, including proton pump inhibitors that provide nearly complete suppression of gastric acid secretion and cytoprotective agents that enhance mucosal defense. The net result is that the prognosis of a patient with peptic acid disease has changed dramatically: medical management can be anticipated to provide a cure, and surgery is only rarely required. The explosive change brought about by the multiplicity of therapeutic tools available for the treatment of patients with peptic acid disease, together with the complexity of the underlying gastrointestinal anatomy and physiology, provided the rationale for the preparation of this monograph.

Our goal in preparing this volume was to contribute to the education of medical students and house staff. The first chapter provides an overview of the anatomy and physiology of the G.I. tract, including the esophagus, stomach, and duodenum. With a good understanding of anatomy and physiology, it is possible to appreciate the interplay between protective and aggressive factors that may lead to irritation or frank ulceration. As noted above, agents are now available that can inhibit or block the secretion of acid, and other agents exist that coat the mucosa of the G.I. tract, minimizing the destructive effects of pepsin and of acid.

Two features of this monograph distinguish it, we believe, from other texts or sources of educational material. The first relates to the multidisciplinary approach that has been taken; such an approach should make the monograph useful to first-year students studying the anatomy and physiology of the gastrointestinal tract, to second-year students learning pathophysiology and pharmacology, and to students in their clinical years, as well as house officers, mastering therapeutic approaches to the treatment of peptic acid disease. The other aspect of this project that distinguishes it from other material available relating to ulcer disease comes from the availability of the original art prepared by Carol Donner. The figures bring life to the text and enhance the description of a complicated subject.

As the project progressed, our perception of the intended audience also changed. In particular, it is our hope that in addition to being of use to students and house officers, the monograph will find its way into the hands of practicing physicians who want to refresh their understanding or update their knowledge of ulcers and other effects of peptic acid.

Preparation of this monograph was made possible by a generous educational grant from SmithKline Beecham.

S B Martin

Editor

Jose Behar, M.D.

ESOPHAGUS

ANATOMY

Overview

The esophagus is a muscular tube lined with a stratified squamous epithelium. It extends from the pharynx at the level of the sixth cervical vertebra through the posterior mediastinum and diaphragm to the stomach. The esophagus enters the abdomen through the esophageal hiatus of the diaphragm forming a short segment of intra-abdominal esophagus before joining the stomach at the cardia (Figure 1). The junction between esophageal squamous epithelium and gastric columnar mucosa appears as an irregular line called the ora serrata or Z-line (Figure 1). The stratified squamous epithelium consists of a basal layer containing dark basophilic nuclei and layers of squamous cells whose nuclei gradually become less pyknotic and eventually disappear before the luminal border is reached (Figure 2). In addition, at various intervals there are projections of lamina propria into the epithelium forming the so-called dermal pegs, which usually extend for about 50% of the total mucosa. The lamina propria contains mononuclear cells, including lymphocytes and plasma cells, as well as blood vessels and nerve fibers. Beneath the lamina propria are the submucosa and then three distinct layers of muscle cells (Figure 2). The external muscle layer is longitudinal; the middle, in which fibers run along the circumference of the esophagus, is circular; and the innermost layer, or muscularis mucosa, also runs in the direction of its longitudinal axis. The upper third of the esophagus contains striated muscle whereas the lower two thirds consists of smooth muscle (Figure 1). Sphincters are located at both ends of the esophagus and are anatomically distinct from the body of the esophagus (Figure 3). The upper esophageal sphincter (UES) appears to be part of the pharynx; its anatomic components are the cricopharyngeus and the inferior pharyngeal constrictor muscles. The lower esophageal sphincter (LES) can also be anatomically identified as a ring of increased thickness of the circular smooth muscle layer (Figure 3) that angles obliquely upward from the lesser to the greater gastric curvature. This ring is split into two segments, one forming short transverse muscle clasps around the esophagus, and the other forming long, oblique loops to the stomach.

Figure 1 (opposite page). Overview of the anatomy of the human esophagus. The upper third has striated muscle, whereas the lower two thirds has smooth muscle.

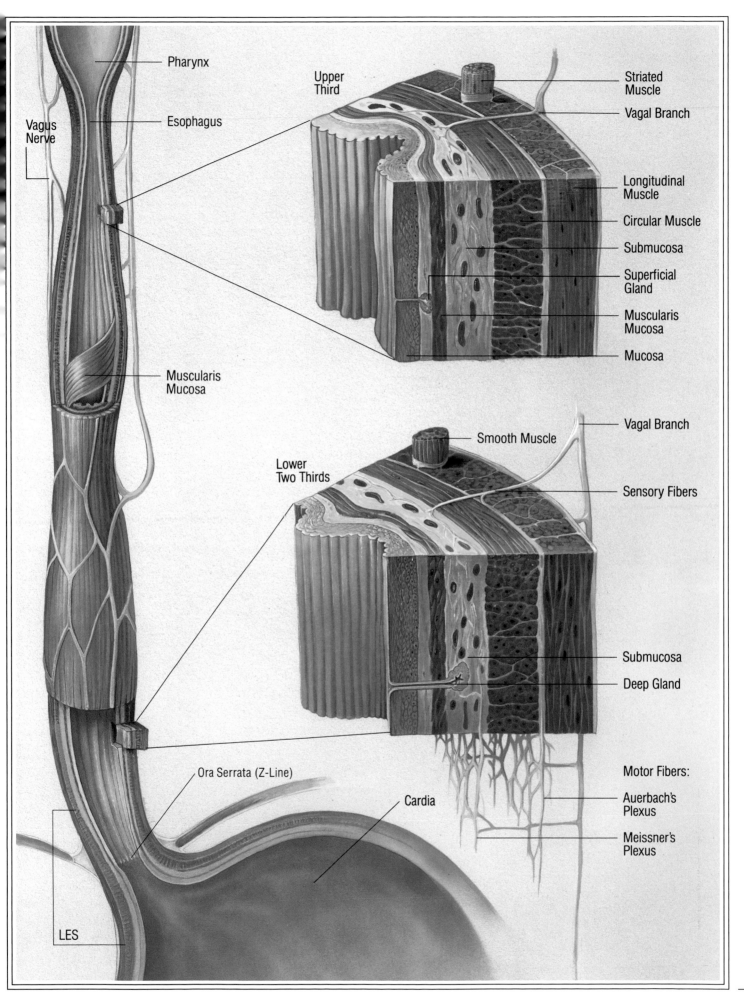

Pharynx

Upper Third

Striated Muscle

Vagal Branch

Vagus Nerve

Esophagus

Longitudinal Muscle

Circular Muscle

Submucosa

Superficial Gland

Muscularis Mucosa

Mucosa

Muscularis Mucosa

Vagal Branch

Smooth Muscle

Sensory Fibers

Lower Two Thirds

Submucosa

Deep Gland

Ora Serrata (Z-Line)

Cardia

Motor Fibers:

Auerbach's Plexus

Meissner's Plexus

LES

2

Figure 1.

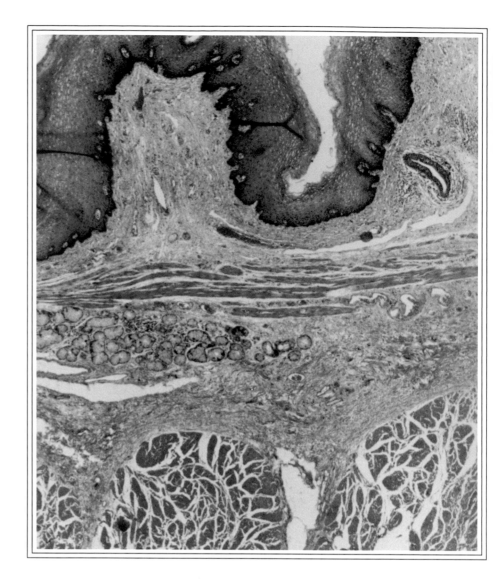

Figure 2. Histology of the esophagus stained with hematoxylin and eosin. The lamina propria is shown in higher power (below). Micrograph provided by S.H. Saul.

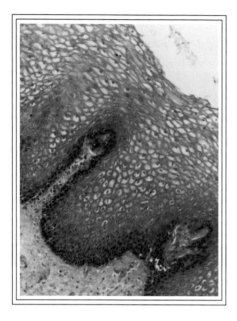

Innervation

The motor innervation of the esophagus arises from the swallowing center located in the brain stem (Figure 4). The vagal fibers that innervate the upper esophageal sphincter and striated muscle segment of the esophagus arise from motor neurons located in the nucleus retrofacialis and the upper neurons of the nucleus ambiguus. These fibers lie within the recurrent laryngeal nerve and innervate individual striated muscle fibers through motor end-plates in a manner similar to somatic innervation elsewhere in the body. The preganglionic fibers that innervate the smooth muscle segment of the esophagus and lower esophageal sphincter arise from the nucleus ambiguus and the dorsal motor nucleus. These preganglionic fibers run in the thoracic branches of the vagus nerve and terminate in the intramural neurons of the enteric nervous system (Figure 4). These vagal fibers are joined by sympathetic fibers that reach the esophagus by way of the perivascular nerves and from splanchnic nerves originating from the celiac ganglia. The sympathetic fibers to the body of the esophagus originate from preganglionic neurons at spinal segments T5 and T6. The intrinsic innervation of the smooth muscle in the lower two thirds of the esophagus consists of numerous ganglion cells and axons and is present in the myenteric (Auerbach's) and submucosal (Meissner's) plexuses (Figure 4).

Figure 3 (opposite page). Anatomy of the upper esophageal sphincter which consists of the inferior constrictor and cricopharyngeal muscles; and, of the lower esophageal sphincter characterized by a thickening of the circular muscle.

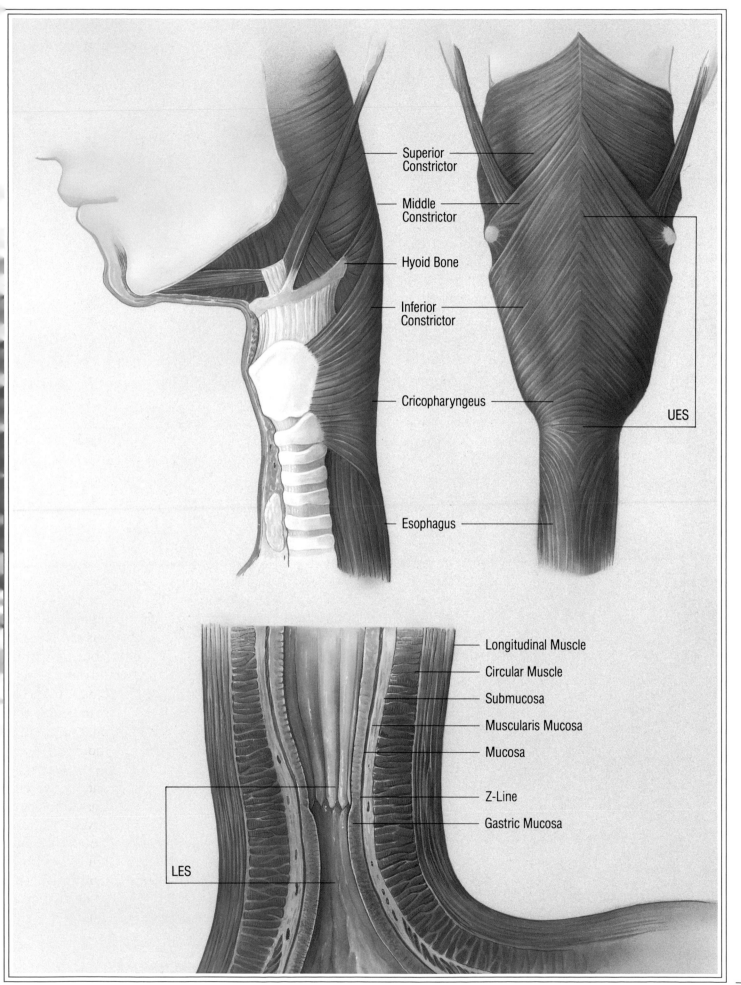

Superior Constrictor

Middle Constrictor

Hyoid Bone

Inferior Constrictor

Cricopharyngeus

UES

Esophagus

Longitudinal Muscle

Circular Muscle

Submucosa

Muscularis Mucosa

Mucosa

Z-Line

Gastric Mucosa

LES

4

Figure 3.

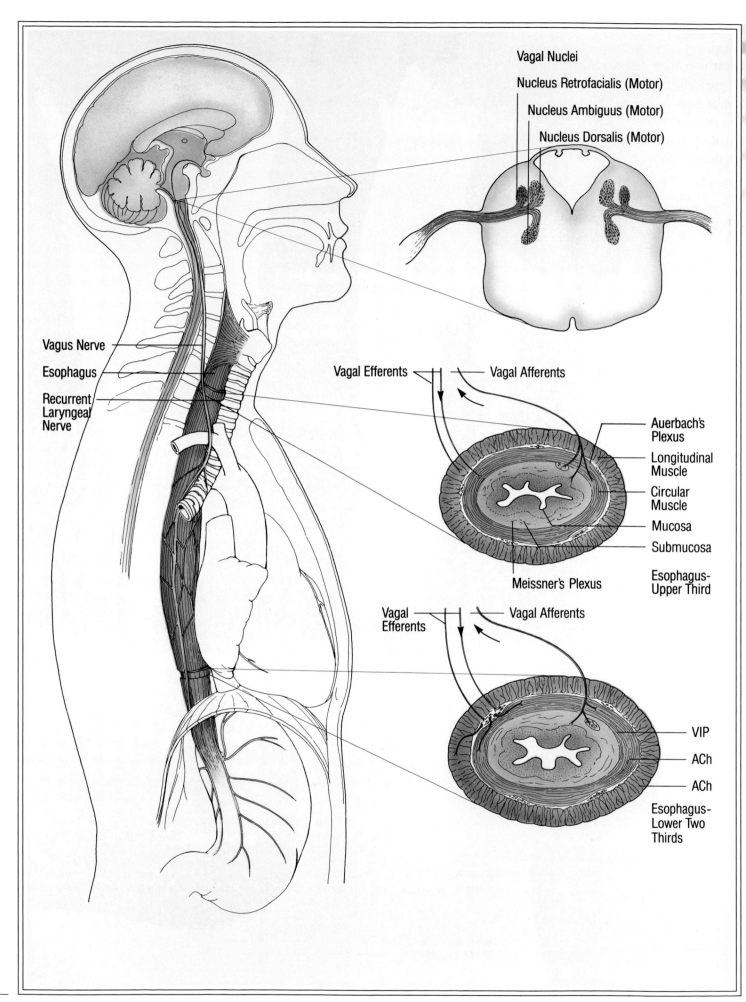

Vagal Nuclei

Nucleus Retrofacialis (Motor)

Nucleus Ambiguus (Motor)

Nucleus Dorsalis (Motor)

Vagus Nerve

Esophagus

Recurrent Laryngeal Nerve

Vagal Efferents — Vagal Afferents

Auerbach's Plexus

Longitudinal Muscle

Circular Muscle

Mucosa

Submucosa

Esophagus-Upper Third

Meissner's Plexus

Vagal Efferents — Vagal Afferents

VIP

ACh

ACh

Esophagus-Lower Two Thirds

Figure 4. Innervation of the esophagus.

The density of the ganglion cells declines from the mid-third of the esophagus to reach a nadir of approximately 100 to 200 cells per square centimeter at the level of the lower esophageal sphincter. Although these cells have not been fully identified morphologically or immunocytochemically, many stain for acetylcholine and for vasoactive intestinal polypeptide (VIP) (Figure 5) as well as for other neuropeptides. There is both sympathetic and parasympathetic innervation of the smooth muscle of the esophagus.

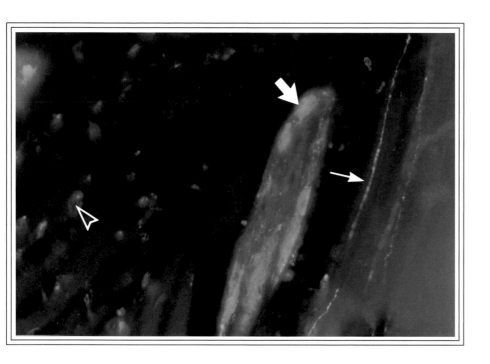

Figure 5. Vasoactive intestinal polypeptide (VIP)-containing cell bodies and axons stained with immunofluorescent techniques. Fibers and cell bodies are seen in the myenteric plexus (bold arrow). Varicosities on fibers (thin arrow) are seen in the longitudinal muscle layer. Fibers in the circular muscle are cut in cross section (open arrowhead). Magnification is approximately 400x. Photograph provided by J.C. Reynolds.

The upper esophageal sphincter is tonically contracted at rest and can be detected manometrically as a zone of high pressure. In humans, the length of this high pressure zone at rest is 2 to 4 cm, with normal pressures varying from 40 to 100 mm Hg above intrathoracic or intraesophageal pressures (Figure 6). The length of the high pressure zone is determined by the cricopharyngeus muscle and the inferior pharyngeal constrictor. Upon deglutition, the UES relaxes fully within 0.2 seconds, with pressures falling to intrathoracic or intraesophageal pressures (Figure 6A, B). This relaxation lasts for approximately 1 second. Sphincter relaxation precedes pharyngeal contraction and thus appears to facilitate the passage of the food bolus. The UES has an additional function of preventing esophago-pharyngeal reflux by responding with reflex contraction to distention or acid perfusion of the upper third of the esophagus.

PHYSIOLOGY

Upper Esophageal Sphincter

Figure 6A. Manometric changes in the pharynx and esophagus evoked by swallowing.

Figure 6B. Comparison of the manometric changes in the pharynx and esophagus induced by swallowing, cervical vagal stimulation and balloon inflation of the mid-esophagus. Secondary peristalsis is evoked following balloon deflation.

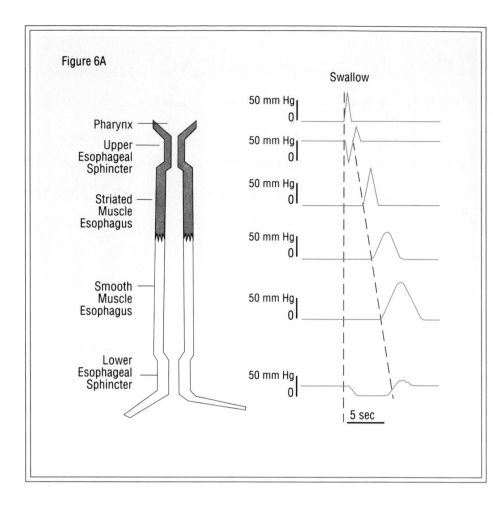

Figure 6A

Peristalsis

Deglutition triggers peristalsis by activating the swallowing center, which initiates an orderly sequential series of contractions from the pharynx through the body of the esophagus to the LES (Figure 6A). There is a very close coordination between the hypopharyngeal, cricopharyngeal, and upper esophageal musculature. In the striated muscle portion of the esophagus, the sequence of the contractions is controlled by a preprogramed reflex in the swallowing center. In the smooth muscle portion of the esophagus, peristalsis is initiated and probably coordinated by the swallowing center and vagus nerves but is primarily controlled by peripheral mechanisms (intramural neurons). Unlike the peristaltic sequences initiated by swallowing, electrical stimulation of the cervical vagus nerve results in simultaneous contraction of the striated muscle in the upper third of the esophagus and relaxation of the UES (Figure 6B). Swallowing and vagal stimulation produce sequential peristaltic contractions in the smooth muscle making up the lower two thirds of the esophagus (Figure 6B). The peristaltic wave travels down the smooth muscle portion of the esophagus at a speed of 3 to 5 cm per second.

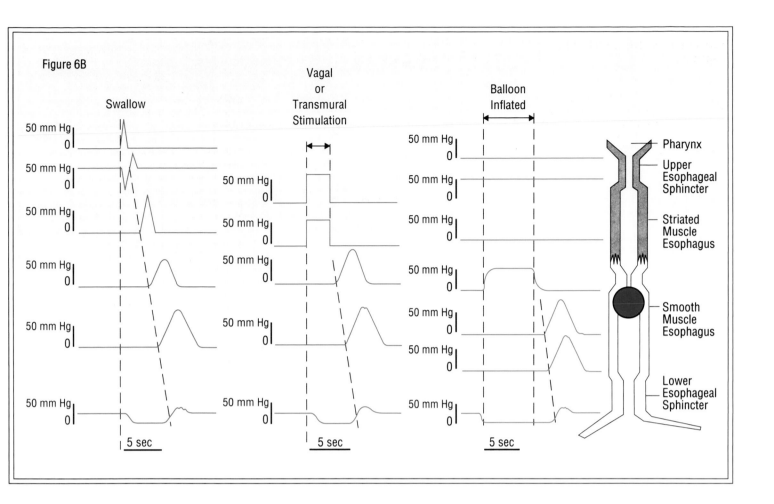

Figure 6B

Primary peristalsis is induced by swallowing whereas secondary peristalsis is initiated by localized esophageal distention by a bolus of food under physiological conditions or by inflation of a small balloon experimentally (Figure 6B). The mechanisms that control secondary peristalsis are also different, depending on whether it is induced in the striated muscle or smooth muscle portion of the esophagus. In the upper third of the esophagus (striated muscle), secondary peristalsis can be induced by distention only if the afferent and efferent extrinsic nerves are intact. In the smooth muscle portion of the esophagus, secondary peristalsis due to esophageal distention can take place in the absence of extrinsic nerves (Figure 6B), indicating that intramural mechanisms can mediate this response.

Lower Esophageal Sphincter

At rest the lower esophageal sphincter maintains a high pressure zone between 15 and 30 mm Hg above intragastric pressures (Figure 6A, B). Swallowing causes relaxation of the LES within 2 seconds, with the effect lasting from 3 to 5 seconds (Figure 6A, B). Full relaxation of the LES precedes esophageal contraction and allows the passage of a food bolus through the LES (Figure 6A, B).

The tonic contraction of the LES is predominantly dependent on myogenic mechanisms of the circular muscle. This muscle is functionally specialized and capable of developing tone in the absence of neural input. LES relaxation induced by swallowing is mediated by the vagus nerve, which synapses with intramural non-adrenergic, non-cholinergic inhibitory fibers. These postganglionic neurons appear to utilize VIP as a neurotransmitter (Figure 7).

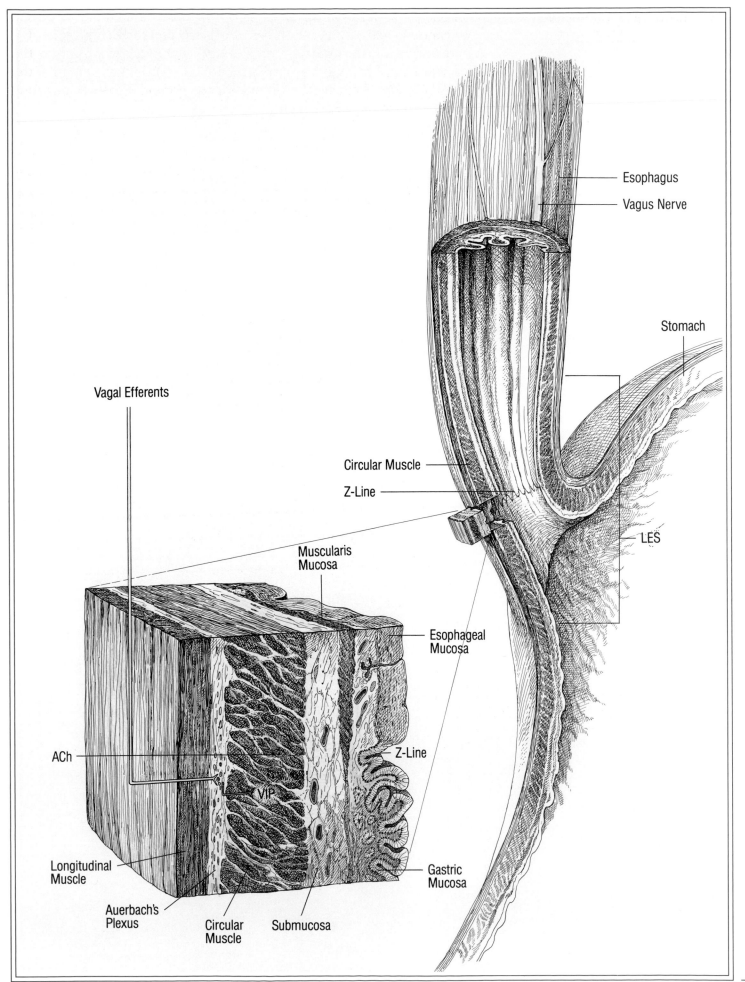

Esophagus

Vagus Nerve

Stomach

Vagal Efferents

Circular Muscle

Z-Line

LES

Muscularis
Mucosa

Esophageal
Mucosa

ACh

Z-Line

VIP

Longitudinal
Muscle

Gastric
Mucosa

Auerbach's
Plexus

Circular
Muscle

Submucosa

Figure 7. Anatomy and neural control of the lower esophageal sphincter.

STOMACH
ANATOMY
Overview

The stomach has been subdivided into anatomical and functional regions. Anatomists have recognized three regions: the fundus, proximal to the gastroesophageal junction; the corpus, or body, between the fundus and the incisura; and, the antrum, from the incisura to the pylorus of the duodenum (Figure 8). From the secretory point of view, there are two distinct areas: a primarily exocrine area consisting of the fundus and body that secretes hydrochloric acid (HCl), pepsin, and intrinsic factor, and a mainly endocrine antropyloric area that is the source of gastrin and most likely of somatostatin and gastrin releasing peptide (GRP).

The gastric wall consists of mucosal and submucosal layers and three muscle layers (Figure 8): a longitudinal outer layer, a middle circular layer, and an inner oblique layer. The most prominent layer throughout much of the stomach is that of circular muscle. The oblique layer, however, is more prominent at the level of the cardia and fundus while the longitudinal layer is prominent in the distal two thirds of the stomach. The circular muscle bundles thicken in the pylorus to form proximal and distal muscle bundles ending in a septum of connective tissue, which marks the gastroduodenal junction.

Innervation

The stomach receives its efferent parasympathetic nerve supply from the vagus nerve whose cell bodies are found in the medulla in the floor of the fourth ventricle (Figure 9). The vagal trunks give off gastric and pyloric branches. The sympathetic supply arises from axons of lateral horn cells located between the 6th and the 9th or 10th thoracic segments. They are carried in the thoracic splanchnic nerves to the celiac plexus and ganglia. Postganglionic fibers make their way to the stomach and the duodenum along the various branches of the celiac and superior mesenteric artery. The enteric plexuses, submucosal plexus (Meissner's), and myenteric plexus (Auerbach's) between layers of the muscular coats contain postganglionic sympathetic and preganglionic parasympathetic fibers, afferent fibers, and intrinsic ganglionic cells and their processes. It is unclear, however, whether preganglionic fibers of the vagus nerve or enteric postganglionic fibers innervate the exocrine and endocrine portions of the stomach.

ENDOCRINE STOMACH
Histology

The so-called endocrine stomach is predominantly located in the mucosa of the antral or pyloric region. The pyloric glands contain both mucous and endocrine cells (Figure 10). Though fewer in number, the endocrine cells are of great importance as a source of polypeptide hormones and biogenic amines. It is estimated that there are about 5×10^5 gastrin secretory cells (G cells) per square centimeter in the stomach of a variety of animal species (Figure 11). These cells can be recognized in electron micrographs because of their triangular shape, with microvilli on the luminal side and multiple granules from 150 to 400

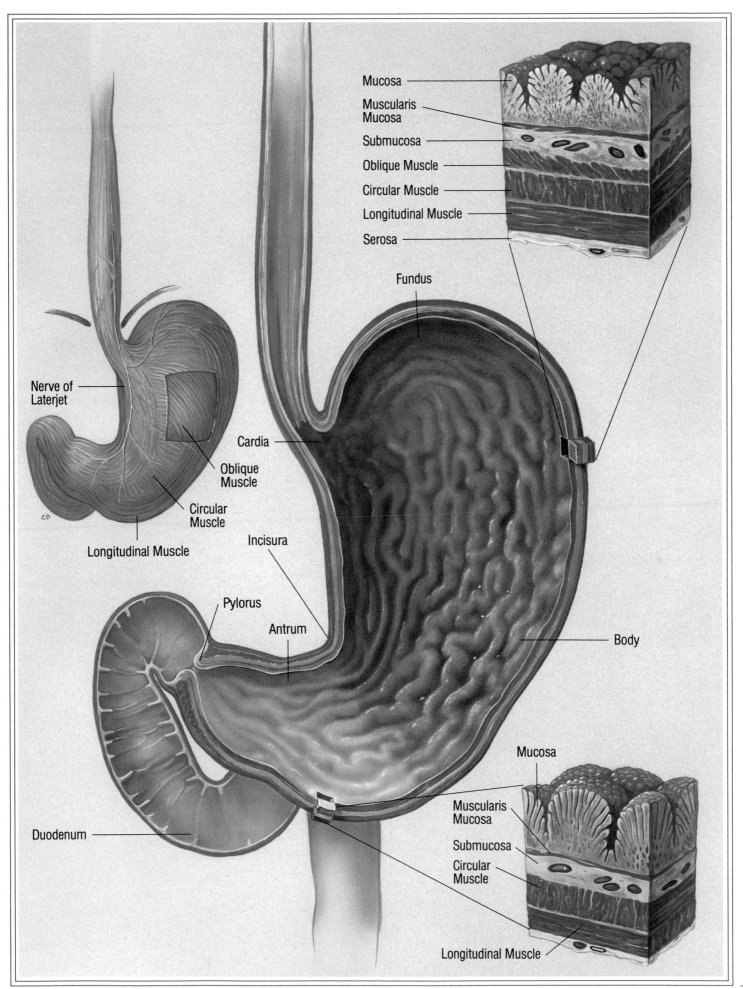

Mucosa

Muscularis
Mucosa

Submucosa

Oblique Muscle

Circular Muscle

Longitudinal Muscle

Serosa

Fundus

Nerve of
Laterjet

Cardia

Oblique
Muscle

Circular
Muscle

Longitudinal Muscle

Incisura

Pylorus

Antrum

Body

Mucosa

Muscularis
Mucosa

Submucosa

Circular
Muscle

Duodenum

Longitudinal Muscle

12

Figure 8. Overview of the anatomy of the stomach.

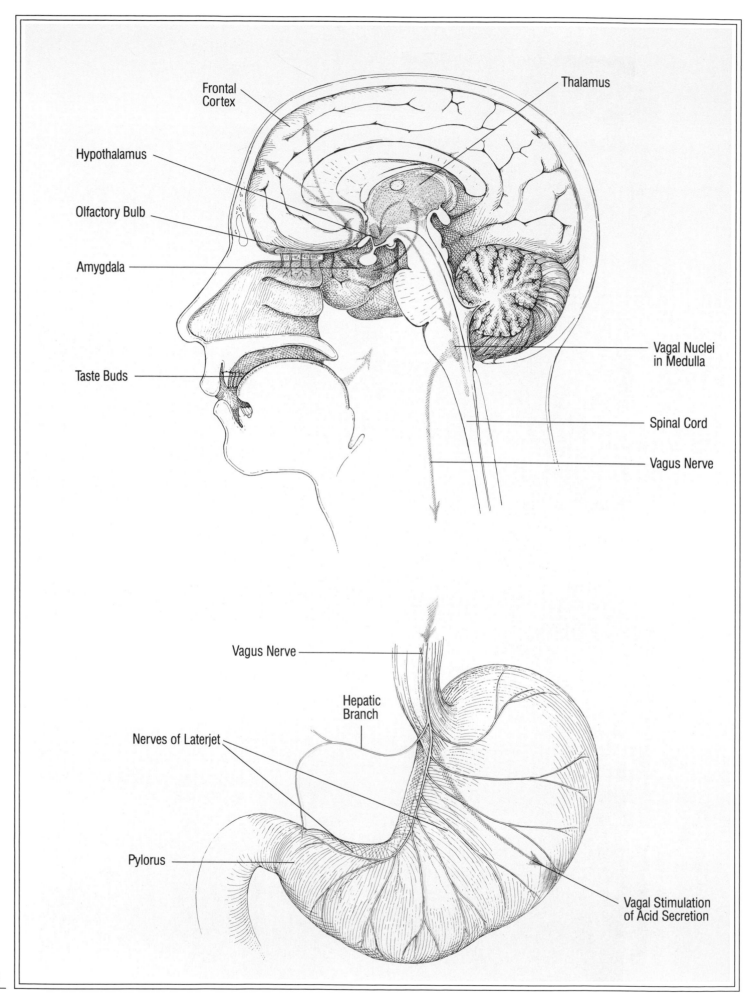

Figure 9. Innervation of the stomach.

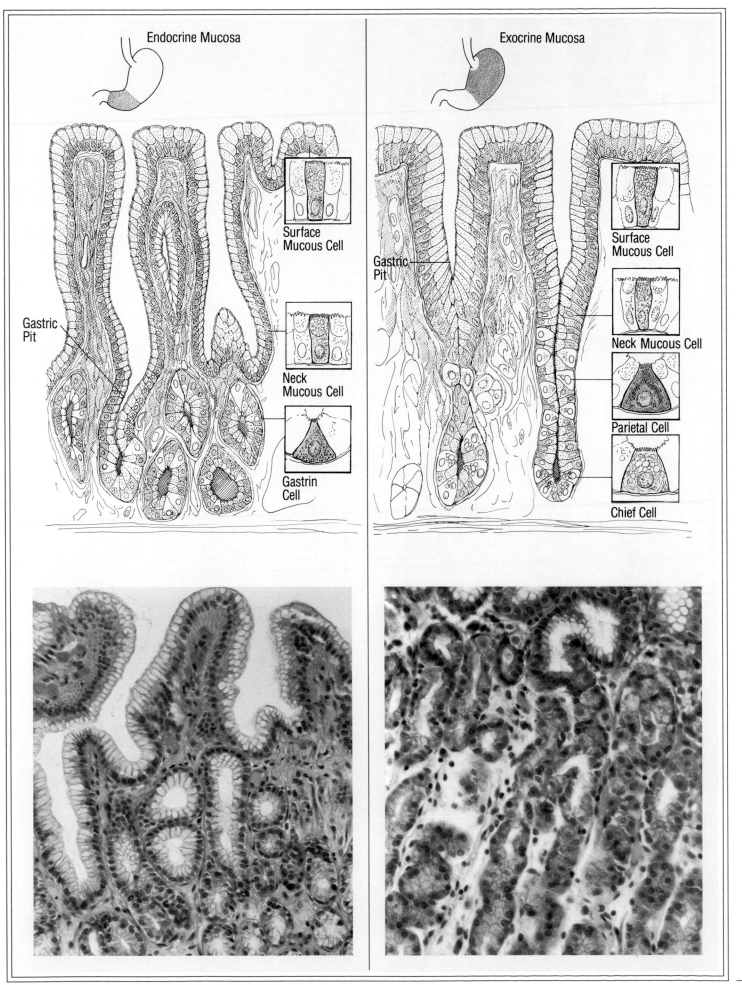

Figure 10. Histology of the gastric mucosa showing the major cell types in the endocrine and exocrine portions of the stomach. Micrographs provided by S.H. Saul.

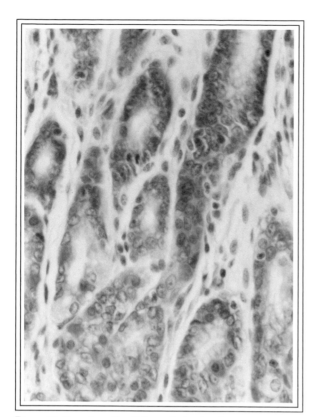

Figure 11. Gastrin cells of the pyloric glands stained with an immunofluorescent technique. Micrograph provided by S.H. Saul.

nanometers in diameter (Figure 12). These granules are storage sites for peptides and are more numerous in the basal cytoplasm. The remaining cytoplasm contains mitochondria and granular endoplasmic reticulum. In humans, G cells do not lie directly on the basal lamina propria but are underlain by processes from neighboring cells, probably from paracrine cells (Figure 13). Other endocrine or paracrine cells in the pyloric mucosa, such as D cells, contain granules that stain for somatostatin. Nerve fibers containing gastrin releasing peptide are also present. In addition, there is evidence for the presence of enterochromaffin cells containing serotonin and histamine.

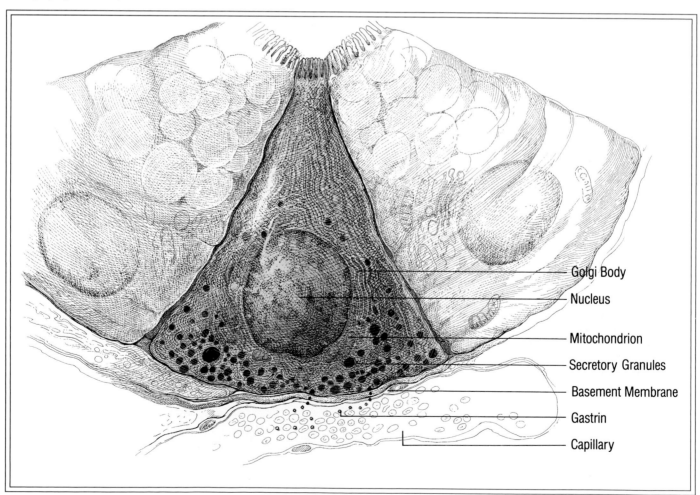

Figure 12. The gastrin cell.

Gastrin is secreted into the circulation in two molecular forms, G-34, which constitutes about two thirds of the gastrin present in fasting subjects, and G-17, the concentration of which increases during the prandial period. It is not known whether basal circulating levels of gastrin come from the antrum or the duodenum. Most of the gastrin released in the stimulated state comes from the antrum. Release of gastrin is stimulated by luminal peptides, amino acids, and calcium; by activation of neuronal reflexes; and by circulating catecholamines and bombesin, or GRP. Phenylalanine and tryptophan are the most potent amino acids regulating the release of gastrin. Feedback inhibition of gastrin release by antral acidification is mediated by regulatory polypeptides including somatostatin and by prostaglandins (Figure 13). Antral acidification inhibits gastrin release when the pH of the gastric lumen falls below 3. On the other hand, alkalinization of the antral lumen does not in and of itself lead to an acute increase in gastrin release. Prolonged neutralization of the stomach contents, as seen in patients with atrophic gastritis, leads to hyperplasia of G cells and to hypergastrinemia.

Gastrin release appears to be under vagal and paracrine control. The effects of the vagus nerve on gastrin release are complex (Figure 13). Activation of vagal cholinergic reflexes by sham feeding or insulin-induced hypoglycemia stimulates the release of gastrin, an effect that can be inhibited by large doses of atropine or antral denervation. In contrast, low doses of atropine enhance the gastrin response to feeding. Basal and postprandial concentrations of gastrin increase after truncal vagotomy. This hypergastrinemia occurs within 48 hours after vagotomy. Cholinomimetic agents cause a weak stimulation of gastrin release but inhibit the increase of gastrin induced by bombesin. Experiments involving selective antral and parietal cell vagotomy reconcile these apparent differences. Gastrin release is mediated by antral vagal fibers, whereas vagal inhibition requires an intact vagal innervation to the proximal stomach. These data are compatible with dual vagal cholinergic mechanisms causing both stimulation and inhibition of gastrin release via separate final pathways and further suggest that hypergastrinemia following vagotomy results from the removal of a predominantly tonic vagal inhibitory mechanism.

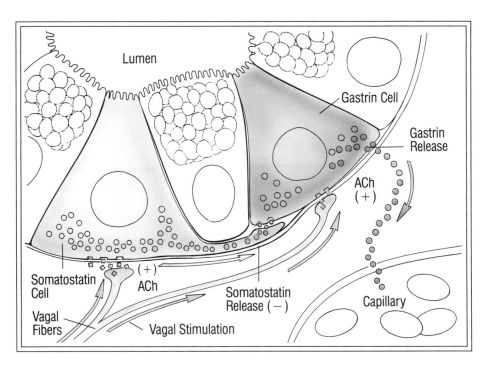

Figure 13. Effects of the vagal innervation of gastrin cells.

There is increasing evidence that somatostatin and gastrin releasing peptide may be the transmitters that mediate these effects. GRP stimulates gastrin release, which may mediate the atropine-resistant, vagally-induced gastrin release. Somatostatin and GRP have been detected in the antral mucosa.

EXOCRINE STOMACH
Histology

The exocrine portion of the stomach corresponds to the fundus and corpus. The entire surface of the glandular stomach is lined by a simple columnar epithelium of surface mucous cells. Scanning electron microscopy of the mucosa reveals a cobblestone surface covered with a blanket of mucous with gastric pits opening at intervals. The gastric pits contain surface mucous cells and neck cells present in the upper third, and large parietal cells and chief cells in the lower two thirds (Figure 10). Chief cells are mostly in the bottom one third of the pits.

Parietal Cells

The parietal cell, which is the most distinct and characteristic gastric cell of the stomach, is the source of hydrochloric acid and intrinsic factor in man. These cells are most numerous in the neck or middle third of the gastric pits, but they are also found in the base of the glands. Histologic preparations have revealed that parietal cells, which stain with acidic dyes such as eosin, are large, oval or pyramidal in shape, and measure about 25 μm in diameter (Figure 14).

In the resting nonsecretory state, parietal cells are filled with tubulovesicular membranes and internalized canaliculi, and they have short microvilli (Figure 14). In the secretory state, the number of intracellular canaliculi is markedly increased, forming a network of canals that may extend into the basal cytoplasm and encircle the nucleus. These canaliculi become externalized, resulting in the formation of long microvilli, which open to the lumen within a larger microvillar surface. There are relatively few tubulovesicular membranes in the cytoplasm while mitochondria appear to occupy about 30% to 40% of the cytoplasmic volume. The microvilli may have a motile function because they have numerous thin filaments containing actin. When active secretion ceases, this motile function may allow withdrawal of the microvillar membrane from the surface into the cytoplasm to reconstitute the tubulovesicular membranes.

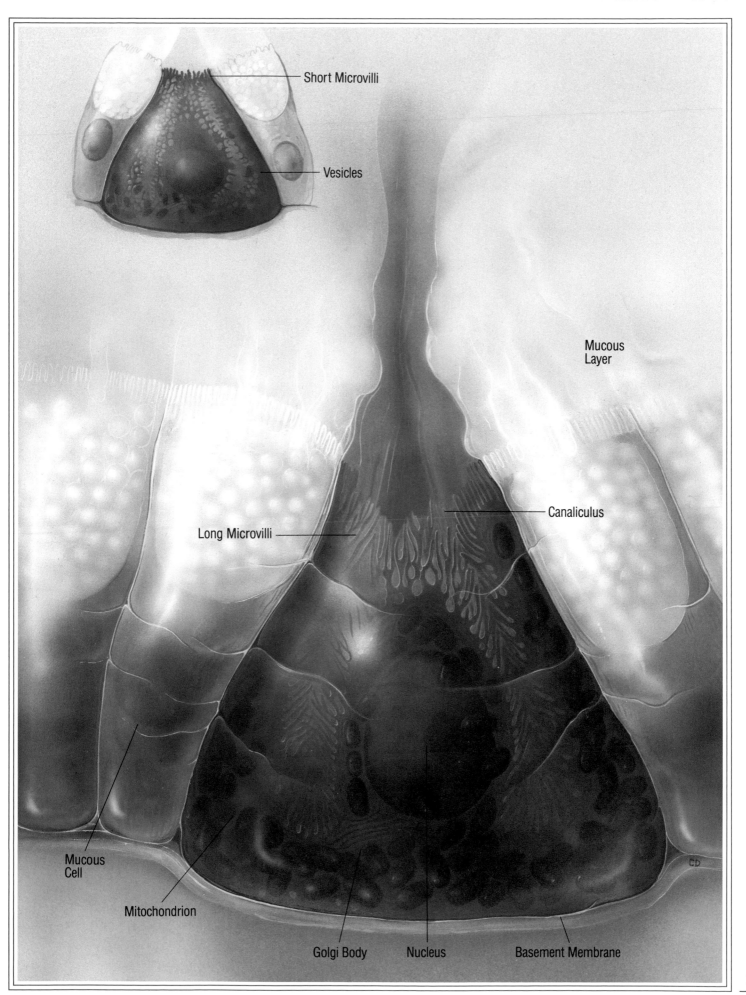

Short Microvilli

Vesicles

Mucous
Layer

Canaliculus

Long Microvilli

Mucous
Cell

Mitochondrion

Golgi Body   Nucleus   Basement Membrane

CD

Figure 14. The parietal cell at rest (top) and after stimulation.

Chief Cells

The chief or peptic cell (Figure 15) is a typical protein-secreting exocrine cell similar in morphology to the pancreatic acinar cell. It synthesizes and stores pepsinogen, the inactive precursor of pepsin. These cells are found predominantly in the base of the gastric pit. Like parietal cells, they are most abundant in the corpus of the stomach. A typical chief cell (Figure 15) is characterized by a luminal surface with short microvilli covered by a thin coating of glycoprotein. Characteristically, they contain zymogen granules, typically 1 to 3 μm in diameter, that store pepsinogen and are usually most numerous in the apical cytoplasm. Pepsinogen is thought to be released by exocytosis or merocrine secretion using similar mechanisms to those involved in secretion of pancreatic zymogen. Studies carried out with fluorescent-labeled antibodies have convincingly demonstrated that chief cells are the primary source of pepsinogen I. Mucous neck cells also appear to contain pepsinogen I, suggesting that two morphologically distinct types of cells may produce this enzyme.

Figure 15. The chief cell.

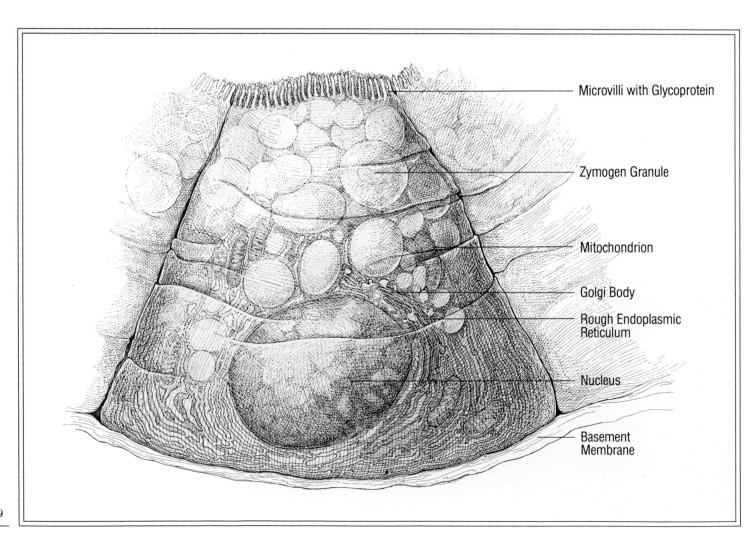

Microvilli with Glycoprotein

Zymogen Granule

Mitochondrion

Golgi Body

Rough Endoplasmic Reticulum

Nucleus

Basement Membrane

There appear to be two types of mucous cells: surface mucous cells that cover the free surface of the glandular stomach and line the upper third of the gastric pits; and neck mucous cells that secrete mucous and resemble intestinal goblet cells (Figure 16). Large numbers of these cells are found in the necks of the gastric pits where they intermingle with parietal cells. Mucous cells also cover the surface of the antral area as well as most of the pyloric glands. The apical part of these cells is packed with mucous-containing granules, and a layer of cytoplasm, rich in web-like filaments, is found in a narrow zone beneath the microvilli and along the lateral cell membrane. The luminal surface of surface mucous cells has short microvilli with a fuzzy surface coat of fine filaments. The major difference between the mucous neck cell and the surface mucous cell is that neck cells stain more deeply with alcian blue at low pH than do surface cells, indicating the presence of more acidic staining sites (mucin) in these cells. Stem cells are also found in the gastric glands. These cells constantly replace gastric epithelium, leading to the formation of mucous neck and surface cells, and oxyntic cells. Mitoses are occasionally observed in these cells.

Proliferation of mucous cells is characteristically rapid. Surface mucous cells are replaced within 3 days, neck mucous cells within 1 week, and parietal, chief, and endocrine cells somewhat more slowly.

Mucous Cells

Figure 16. Mucous-secreting cell.

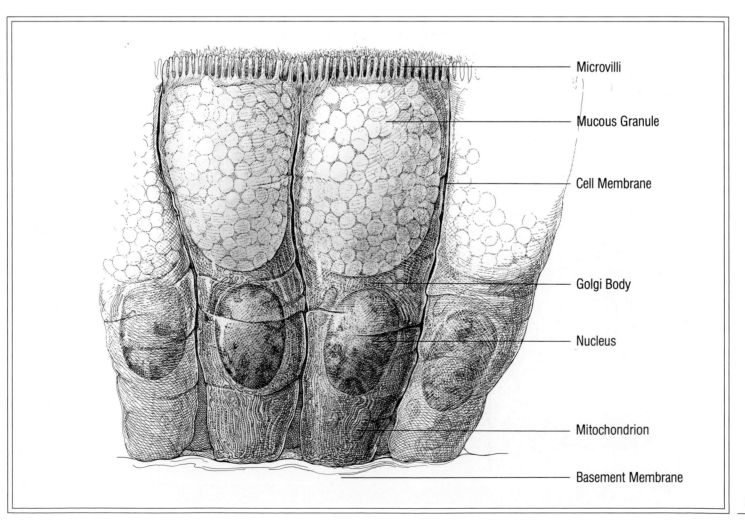

Microvilli

Mucous Granule

Cell Membrane

Golgi Body

Nucleus

Mitochondrion

Basement Membrane

Basal Secretion: Basal gastric acid secretion takes place in the fasting state (Figure 17). This secretion shows a circadian rhythm, with high rates in the evening and low rates in the morning. It is mainly dependent on the vagus nerve and basal secretion is markedly reduced following abdominal vagotomy. The release of gastrin, which probably plays a minor role, is secondary to tonic vagal activity.

Prandial Secretion: Acid secretion in the prandial state includes excitatory and inhibitory neurohormonal mechanisms that turn acid secretion on and off as the meal is transported from the oral cavity to the small intestine.

Cephalic phase: Secretion takes place in response to the association, perception, or chewing of food. It is initiated by the sight or smell of food, by association with the thought of food (Figure 18), and in the laboratory it has been shown that "sham feeding" during which food is chewed but not swallowed causes an increase in acid secretion. In humans, sham feeding can stimulate about 40% of the maximal secretory response to pentagastrin, whereas in the dog it can maximally stimulate acid secretion. This cephalic phase can also be triggered by hypoglycemia. Vagal stimulation activates gastric acid secretion by direct action on the parietal cells and indirectly by stimulating the release of gastrin from the antrum. However, gastrin plays a minor role in this phase of acid secretion. Antrectomy reduces the acid response to sham feeding, probably as a result of interrupting the innervation to the remaining pouch. The response to exogenous pentagastrin is also reduced by 50% by antrectomy, and the acid response to sham feedings is not restored by infusion of pentagastrin.

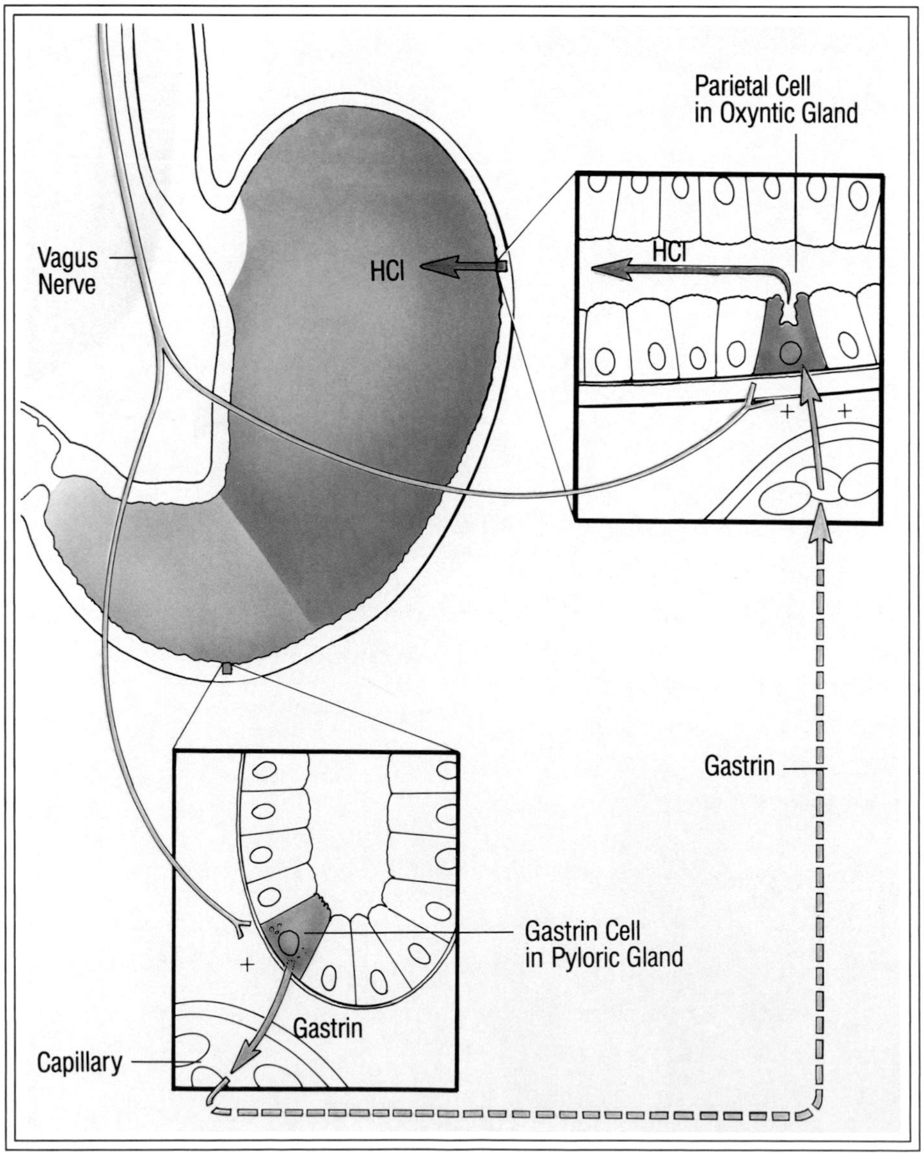

Figure 17. Control of fasting acid secretion.

An inhibitory component of the cephalic phase has been postulated to exist. This hypothesis is supported by studies with experimental animals in which injection of peptides, including bombesin, GRP, or corticotropin releasing factor (CRF), into either the cisterna magna or the lateral cerebral ventricle causes inhibition of gastric acid secretion. The inhibitory action of CRF is abolished by truncal vagotomy.

Gastric phase: The excitatory pathways of this phase are triggered by the presence of food in the stomach, which influences gastric acid secretion through mechanical distention and chemical mechanisms. The effects of distention are mediated by vagal mechanisms and by gastrin. The neural mechanisms are mediated by long vago-vagal and short intramural reflexes. Gastrin release can be prevented by antral acidification, whereas a vago-vagal reflex (pyloro-oxyntic reflex) is abolished only by vagal denervation of the antral pouch (Figure 19).

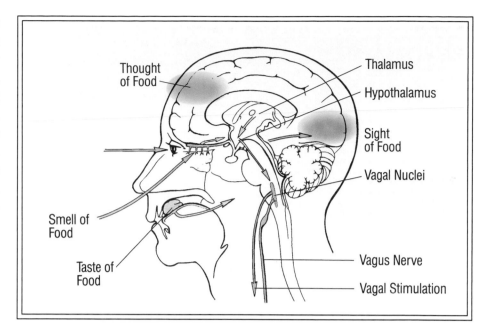

Figure 18. Cephalic phase of acid secretion.

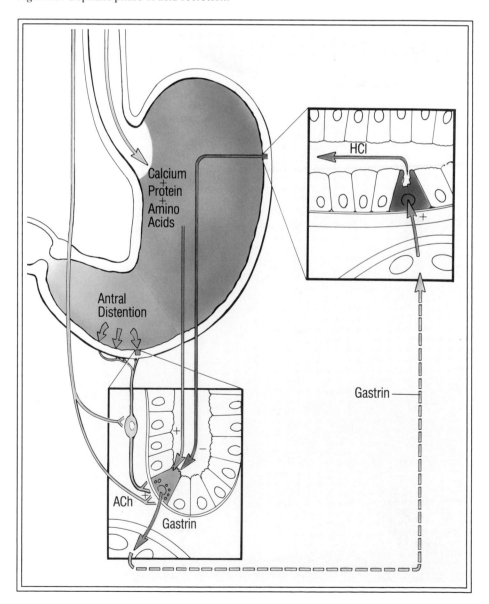

Figure 19. Gastric phase of acid secretion.

Distention of the intact dog stomach by food stimulates moderate rates of secretion by mechanisms that do not involve the release of gastrin. Graded distention of a vagally innervated antral pouch leads to stepwise increases in serum gastrin concentration and in acid secretion from a vagally innervated gastric fistula. This increase in gastric secretion induced by antral distention involves at least two mechanisms: 1) gastrin release, which can be prevented by acidification; and 2) a vago-vagal reflex (pyloro-oxyntic reflex), which is abolished by vagal denervation of the antral pouch.

Chemical agents, including caffeine, alcohol, calcium, and products of protein digestion, are among the regularly ingested substances known to stimulate acid secretion. These substances appear to cause an incremental increase in secretion of gastrin and acid.

Inhibitory pathways are activated by antral acidification, which blocks release of gastrin induced by sham feeding, antral distention, and chemical stimulation. Marked suppression is seen at a pH of 2, and complete abolition of acid secretion is seen at a pH of 1.

Intestinal phase: The entry of food into the duodenum can stimulate gastric acid secretion. Initiators of this phase are, as in the stomach, distention and products of protein digestion, including peptides and amino acids. The mediators of this phase are in part humoral because acid secretion is not abolished by denervation. It is likely that gastrin plays an important role. It is unclear, however, whether the release of gastrin is due to luminal effects or to systemic stimulation after amino acids have been absorbed. Intravenously administered amino acids stimulate gastric acid secretion, and infusion of amino acids into the duodenum results in an increase in the release of gastrin (Figure 20).

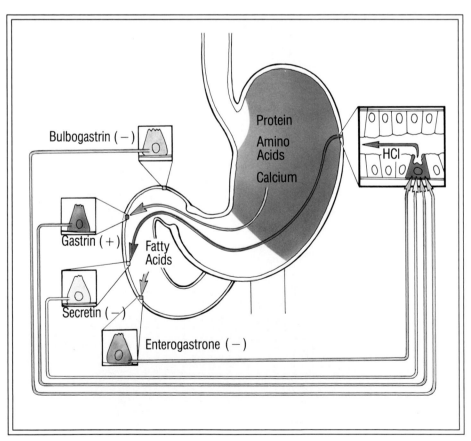

Figure 20. Intestinal phase of acid secretion.

The intestinal phase, however, is predominantly inhibitory, as gastric contents entering the small intestine elicit neurohormonal mechanisms that turn off acid secretion. Acid, fat, and hyperosmolar solutions, when infused into the duodenum and small intestine, inhibit acid secretion. Acid probably inhibits acid secretion via an effect on the release of secretin: 1) acid and exogenous secretin inhibit pentagastrin-stimulated acid secretion but are ineffective against histamine-stimulated secretion; 2) graded rates of acid infusion cause graded increases in pancreatic bicarbonate secretion and graded decreases in acid secretion; and, 3) acid and exogenous secretin-induced inhibition of acid release appear to be noncompetitive. However, when acid is confined to the duodenal bulb, gastric acid secretion is reduced by mechanisms that do not involve secretin since pancreatic bicarbonate secretion is not affected. This acid-induced inhibition may be mediated by a still unidentified hormone called bulbogastrone.

Fat also inhibits acid secretion, after being converted to absorbable fatty acids or monoglycerides. This effect is mediated by humoral mechanisms involving a still unidentified hormone called enterogastrone (Figure 20). Three candidates have been proposed: gastric inhibitory polypeptide, neurotensin, and peptide YY. Although all three hormones are released in response to the presence of fat in the small intestine, and all decrease acid secretion, none completely mimics the inhibitory effect of fat. Neurotensin appears to be the strongest candidate because it is released by fat from the distal intestine and it inhibits pentagastrin-stimulated acid secretion.

Secretion of acid from parietal cells:

Stimulation: Parietal cells are stimulated by three secretagogues: acetylcholine, a neurotransmitter released from the vagus nerve; the paracrine substance histamine; and the hormone gastrin. Although parietal cells have receptors for all three secretagogues (Figure 21A), the finding that specific H_2 blockers not only antagonize histamine-induced secretion but also acetylcholine and gastrin-stimulated secretion are consistent with the view that acetylcholine and gastrin may stimulate parietal cells indirectly by releasing histamine from paracrine cells (Figure 21B).

Figure 21 A and B. Models of possible mechanisms of parietal cell stimulation by acetylcholine, histamine, and gastrin.

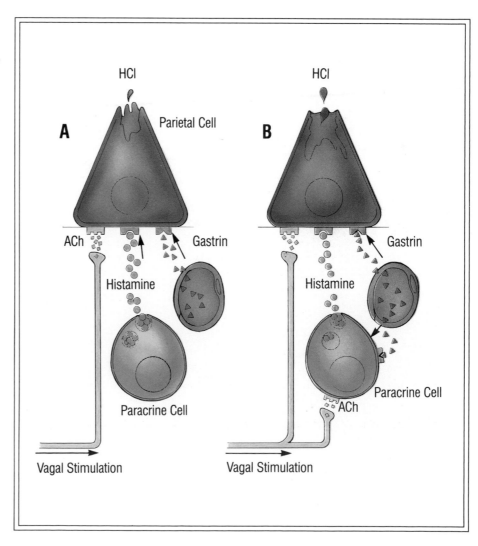

Intracellular Mechanisms: Histamine, acting through H_2 receptors, causes an increase in intracellular levels of cyclic AMP (Figure 22). Effects of acetylcholine and gastrin are mediated through increases in cytosolic calcium. Acetylcholine increases calcium influx from the extracellular space while gastrin may mobilize calcium from intracellular stores. Increases in cellular cyclic AMP levels or in free cytosolic calcium result in the activation of one or more protein kinases and in the phosphorylation of a variety of proteins that activate the intracellular secretory canaliculi (Figure 22).

Formation of Secretory Canaliculi: Stimulation of receptors on parietal cells increases cellular cyclic AMP levels and/or free cytosolic calcium, which, through activation of one or more protein kinases, activates the canaliculi with morphologic and functional consequences (Figure 22).

Figure 22. Activation of the parietal cell.

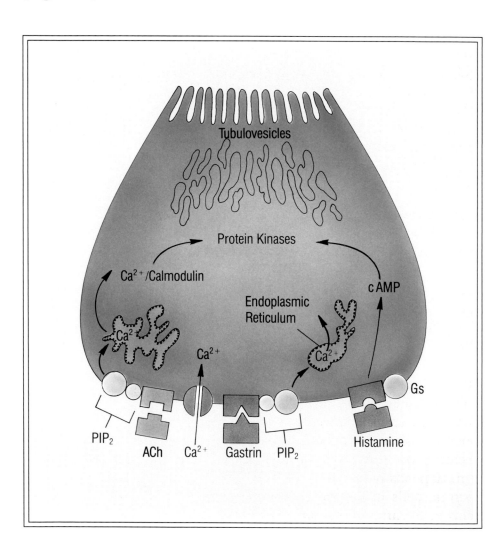

The canaliculi become externalized after fusing to the apical membrane, forming long microvilli opening into the lumen. The increase in second messengers induces the movement of a hydrogen-potassium ATPase from the tubulovesicles into the secretory canaliculi. This enzyme promotes electrogenic entry of potassium and chloride (Figure 23). Entry 7f potassium into the secretory canaliculi is required for the hydrogen pump [H^+/K^+—ATPase] to cause the electroneutral exchange of hydrogen for potassium in the presence of ATP and magnesium. The electrogenic entry of potassium and chloride appears to operate in parallel to the ATP-driven hydrogen-potassium exchange pump. The net effect is the rapid accumulation of hydrochloric acid within the vesicles. Hydrogen is generated by dissociation of water into hydrogen (H^+) and hydroxyl (OH^-) ions that takes place in the presence of the enzyme carbonic anhydrase and results in the formation of carbonic acid. A carbonic acid-chloride exchange (HCO_3/Cl) occurs at the basolateral membrane, which provides the necessary chloride on a 1:1 basis for each hydrogen (Figure 23). Cellular potassium levels are maintained, in part, by the Na^+/K^+— ATPase also present in the basolateral membrane, and the internal sodium requirement is, in part, satisfied by the sodium-hydrogen (Na^+/H^+) exchange. The overall efficiency of the process is remarkable since the pH of the cell is only slightly above the resting level of 7.2.

Each active parietal cell is thought to generate acid at the same rate, so that the major variable determining total output is the number of parietal cells secreting at any one time. In the basal state, only a few parietal cells secrete acid; during a meal or after the administration of an exogenous secretagogue, increasing numbers of cells are stimulated to secrete acid. The maximal ability of the stomach to secrete acid and the secretory response to stimulation by a maximally effective dose of a secretagogue (histamine or pentagastrin) depends on the total number of oxyntic cells in the gastric mucosa. This is, in turn, a function of parietal cell mass. It has been estimated that stomachs of normal subjects contain about a billion parietal cells. This increase in gastric secretory rates is accompanied by a marked increase in hydrogen ion concentration and to a lesser extent in chloride concentration (Figure 24).

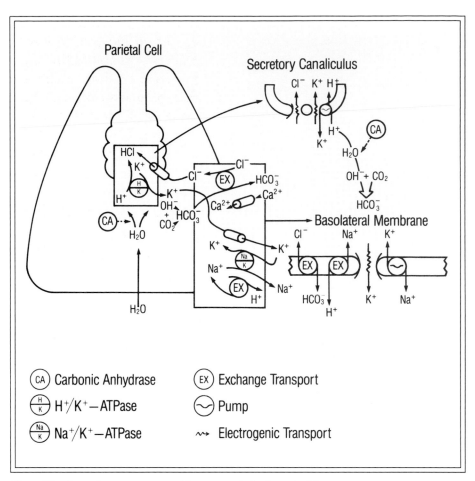

Figure 23. Electrolyte transport and homeostasis in the apical (secretory canaliculus) and basolateral membranes of the parietal cell.

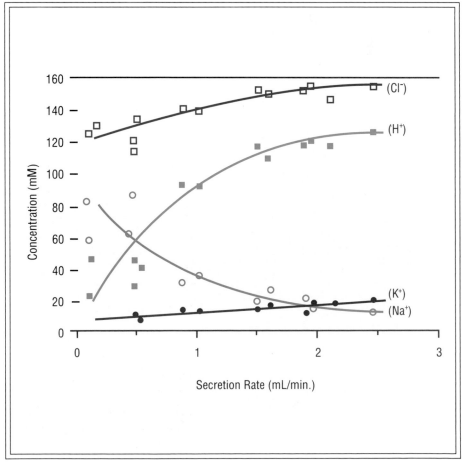

Figure 24. Relationship between electrolyte concentration and secretion rate. Adapted from Nordgren, *Acta Physiol Scandinav*, 1963;58(Suppl. 202):1-83.

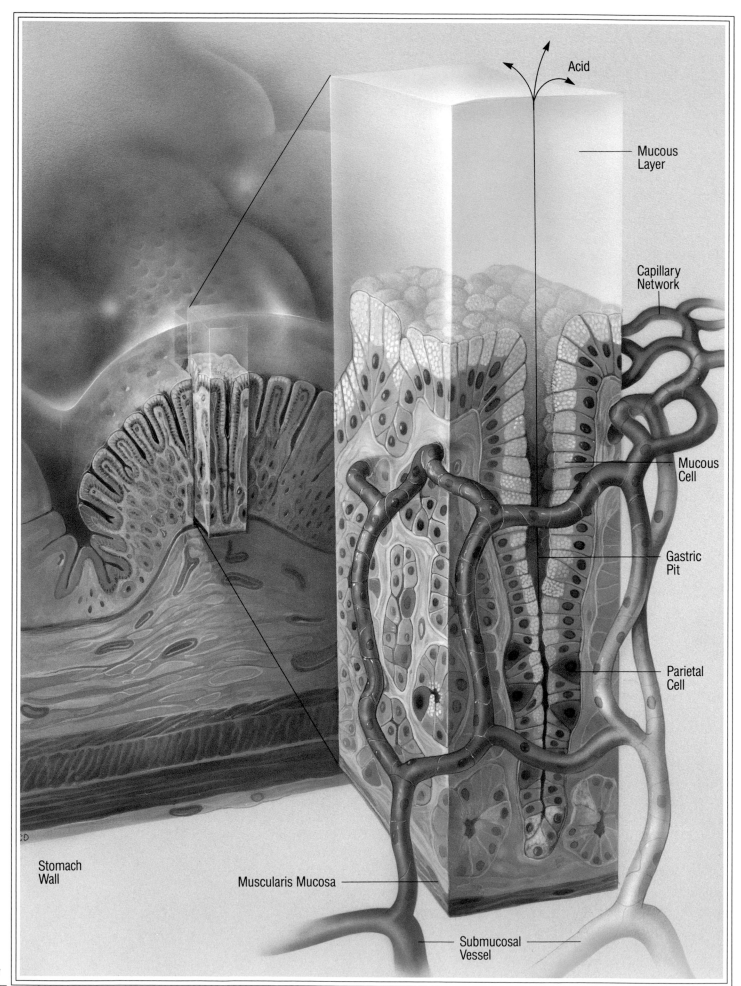

Acid

Mucous
Layer

Capillary
Network

Mucous
Cell

Gastric
Pit

Parietal
Cell

Stomach
Wall

Muscularis Mucosa

Submucosal
Vessel

27

Figure 25. Blood supply to the gastric mucosa.

Stimulation of gastric acid secretion is accompanied by increases in blood supply to the gastric mucosa (Figure 25). Increased blood flow is a permissive physiological event because adequate flow is necessary for the stomach to secrete acid. Profound vasoconstriction caused by sympathetic stimulation following administration of vasoactive drugs is followed by depression of acid secretion. Increased blood flow in itself does not result, however, in stimulation of acid secretion.

Pepsinogen, initially formed as prepepsinogen, is secreted into the lumen, and, under acidic conditions between pH 5 and 2, gradually converted into pepsin, the active form of the enzyme (Figure 26). The transformation of pepsinogen into pepsin results from removal of the amino terminal signal peptide. Since pepsinogen has no catalytic activity, it is measured by radioimmunoassay. Such techniques have led to identification of two immunoreactive pepsinogens: pepsinogen I, secreted by chief cells and, to a limited extent, by mucous neck cells, and pepsinogen II, secreted by mucous cells of the gastrointestinal tract. Results of recent studies have improved our understanding of the neurohormonal mechanisms controlling secretion of pepsinogen. Pepsinogen secretion is under vagal control. Acetylcholine, released from the nerve, activates a muscarinic receptor, an effect that is blocked by atropine or pirenzepine. Secretion of pepsinogen is also stimulated by gastrointestinal hormones, including CCK and gastrin, by neuropeptides, including VIP, and by histamine and isoproterenol. These stimuli activate two different intracellular effector systems in chief cells. CCK and gastrin appear to stimulate the hydrolysis of phosphatidylinositol, resulting in an increase in cytosolic calcium and activation of protein kinase C. Histamine, secretin, VIP, and isoproterenol stimulate pepsinogen secretion by activating adenyl cyclase, leading to an increase in intracellular levels of cyclic AMP and activation of cyclic AMP dependent protein kinase.

The major physiologic function of pepsin is initiation of protein digestion. The quantitative contribution of pepsin to the overall digestive process is probably minor. The proteolytic activity of pepsin is of brief duration since gastric contents are rapidly buffered. Pepsin is highly active on collagen and is probably more important for the digestion of meat than vegetable protein. In general, protein is broken down into large peptides that normally enter the intestine before digestion is complete.

Intrinsic factor: The parietal cell is the source of intrinsic factor in man. The amount of intrinsic factor secreted greatly exceeds the amount needed to bind vitamin B-12 (cobalamin). Cobalamin in turn is essential for normal division and viability of cells, but it is not synthesized in mammalian cells. The neurohormonal mechanisms that control synthesis and secretion of intrinsic factor are similar to those that control acid secretion (Figure 27). Histamine increases the release of intrinsic factor through mechanisms involving stimulation of the synthesis of cyclic AMP.

Pepsinogen Secretion

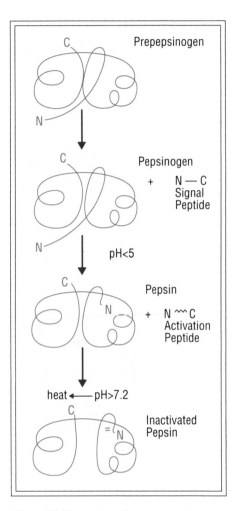

Figure 26. Formation of active pepsin. Adapted from Tang, *Mole Cell Biochem,* 1979;26(2):93-109. Andreeva, et al, *Biochem Biophys Res Comm,* 1979;87(1):32-42.

Other Secretions

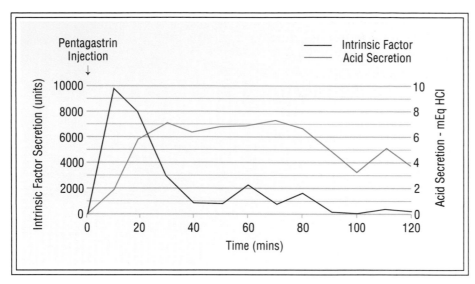

Figure 27. Release of acid and intrinsic factor by gastrin. Gastrin (6 units/kg) was administered at time zero. Adapted from Donaldson, in *Physiology of the Gastrointestinal Tract*, 1987.

Intrinsic factor is a globular glycoprotein, with a molecular weight of about 44,000 Daltons, 15% of which is carbohydrate. It has a high affinity for vitamin B-12. The configuration of the intrinsic factor molecule changes when it binds to cobalamin, becoming more compact. The complex of intrinsic factor-cobalamin is more resistant to proteases than is free intrinsic factor. Humans need to absorb about 1 to 2 μg of vitamin B-12 daily to maintain normal hepatic stores.

The transport and absorption of cobalamin follows a well understood sequence. First, cobalamin is released from dietary protein as a consequence of the action of acid and pepsin in the stomach. It is then bound tightly to salivary proteins called R proteins (Figure 28A). When the cobalamin-R protein complex enters the duodenum, the R protein is digested by pancreatic proteases, which again release cobalamin. At this point, intrinsic factor binds cobalamin (Figure 28A). This binding appears to be very specific since intrinsic factor has a low affinity for analogues of cobalamin. The intrinsic factor-cobalamin complex is transported down the intestine to the ileum where, in the presence of calcium, this complex attaches to the absorptive surface of the ileal columnar cells. Then the entire complex enters the cell where intrinsic factor appears to release cobalamin, which is then bound to transcobalamin, either within the cell or at the serosal side of the cell (Figure 28B).

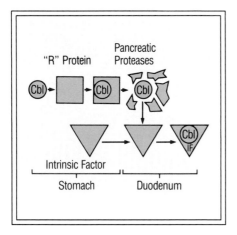

Figure 28A.

Mucous secretion: Mucous cells (Figure 16) synthesize glycoproteins in the golgi complex. It has been suggested that release of mucous takes place by exocytosis, apical expulsion, or cell exfoliation. Exocytosis of mucous granules appears to be a slow but continuous process in contrast to the sudden release of all the stored mucous during apical expulsion, which is followed by cell degeneration. A final method, rarely observed, is the exfoliation of the entire cell. The last two forms of mucous secretion tend to occur mainly on the surface but not in the gastric pits.

Bicarbonate secretion: Surface mucous cells appear to be the major source of bicarbonate secretion in the stomach. These cells have high levels of carbonic anhydrase, the enzyme responsible for carbonic acid formation. An additional source of bicarbonate appears to involve the uptake of carbonic acid released by the oxyntic cells into the circulation during acid formation. Bicarbonate secretion is stimulated by a number of neurotransmitters, hormones, and autacoids, including acetylcholine, CCK, neurotensin, pancreatic glucagon, prostaglandins of the E and F_2 alpha series, cyclic GMP, and calcium.

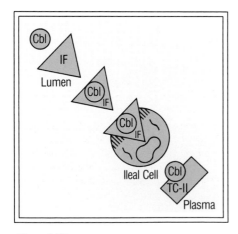

Figure 28B.

Figure 28A and B. Absorption of cobalamin (cbl). The rules of intrinsic factor (IF) and transcobalamin 11 (TC-11) are shown.

Secretion of bicarbonate is inhibited by atropine, inhibitors of cyclo-oxygenase such as indomethacin, as well as by ethanol, taurocholate, and acetozolamide. Neither gastrin nor histamine seems to have any effect on the secretion of bicarbonate. In man, sham feeding and cholinergic stimulation increase secretion of bicarbonate, and this effect is inhibited by atropine, suggesting that secretion is under vagal control. It has also been shown that secretion of bicarbonate is stimulated by the cytoprotective action of prostaglandins of the E type and inhibited by compounds that break the gastric mucosal barrier, such as luminal bile and aspirin. Results of *in vitro* studies have led to the conclusion that bicarbonate secretion is an electroneutral process not associated with changes in the transmucosal electrical potential. It is thought to involve an electroneutral chloride/carbonic acid exchange at the luminal cell membrane. High carbonic anhydrase activity is localized in the apical cytoplasmic matrix and microvillar cores.

Gastric Emptying

The stomach empties liquids, solid foods, and indigestible particles at different rates (Figure 29). Emptying of liquids such as dextrose solution initially takes place rapidly, then slows with time. Increasing concentrations of nutrients, acidity, or salts in liquid meals slows gastric emptying. As the solute concentration of a liquid meal increases, the rate of gastric emptying becomes less exponential and more linear. Gastric emptying of solids is somewhat different and follows a sigmoidal curve (Figure 29). There is an initial lag phase during which no solid food is emptied, but solid chyme is converted into smaller fragments and particles, so they may pass through the pyloric sphincter. This lag phase is followed by a more prolonged emptying phase. The effect of the volume of a solid meal on gastric emptying is complex. Increasing the volume tends to accelerate gastric emptying, provided that the caloric content remains constant; however, when there is a concomitant increase in calories and volume, the gastric emptying rate slows because the volume effect is overridden by the inhibition induced by the increased number of calories entering the duodenum. Analysis of a mixed solid/liquid test meal shows that the liquid phase empties more rapidly than the solid phase, which is termed "solid/liquid discrimination." The much slower emptying of indigestible particles seems to indicate that the initial lack in emptying of solids involves more than reducing solids to small particles acceptable by the relaxed pyloric sphincter. Large indigestible particles are emptied mainly during phase III of the inter-digestive cycle, the migrating motor complex.

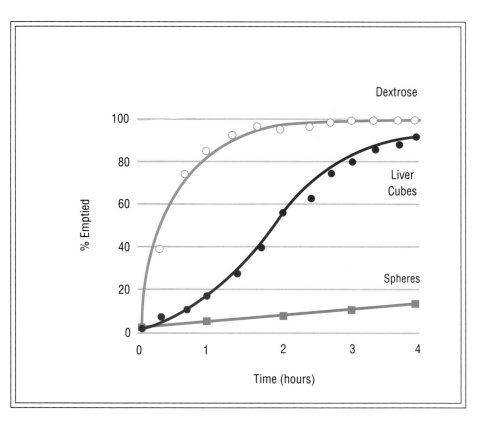

Figure 29. Time-course of gastric emptying of liquids (1% dextrose), solids and indigestible particles (plastic spheres 7 mm in diameter). Adapted from Hinder, et al, *Am J Physiol*, 1977;233(4):E335-E340.

DUODENUM
ANATOMY

The duodenum is a tubular organ comprising the intestinal segment between the end of the pylorus and the ligament of Treitz (Figure 30). It is mostly retroperitoneal, with the exception of the bulb, and has been divided into four portions: the duodenal bulb; the descending portion; the horizontal portion, which crosses transversely anterior to the interior vena cava and aorta; and the ascending portion, which extends toward the ligament of Treitz to become the jejunum. The duodenum has a C-like shape, with the common bile duct and the pancreatic duct draining into the ampulla located in the medial aspect of the mid-portion of the descending duodenum. It consists of five layers: the mucosa; submucosa; two muscular layers, the inner or circular muscle and the outer longitudinal muscle; and the serosa. The duodenum differs from the jejunum in that, at least in the first and second portions, the villi tend to be shorter and somewhat clubbed (Figure 31) and Brunner's glands are found in the submucosa (Figure 32). The duodenum is also innervated by preganglionic parasympathetic fibers that run in the vagus nerve and synapse with intramural neurons.

PHYSIOLOGY
Surface Epithelium

The duodenal mucosa, like the gastric mucosa, secretes mucous and bicarbonate. *In vitro*, bicarbonate secretion is stimulated by prostaglandins, by dibutyryl cyclic AMP, and by hormones, such as gastric inhibitory peptide and pancreatic glucagon; it is inhibited by acetazolamide and inhibitors of cyclo-oxygenase. It is thought that secretion of bicarbonate takes place as a result of a variety of different mechanisms: electroneutral exchange of chloride for bicarbonate occurs at the luminal membrane and is stimulated by hormones and inhibited by furosemide. This transport is stimulated by prostaglandins and cyclic AMP and is ouabain sensitive, suggesting an interaction with the enzyme sodium-potassium ATPase. Another possible mechanism is passive movement of bicarbonate through shunt pathways sensitive to variations in transmucosal hydrostatic pressure. Bicarbonate secretion by the duodenal surface epithelium is also stimulated by beta-endorphins and enkephalins and is unaffected by histamine, serotonin, somatostatin, bombesin, substance P, or taurocholate.

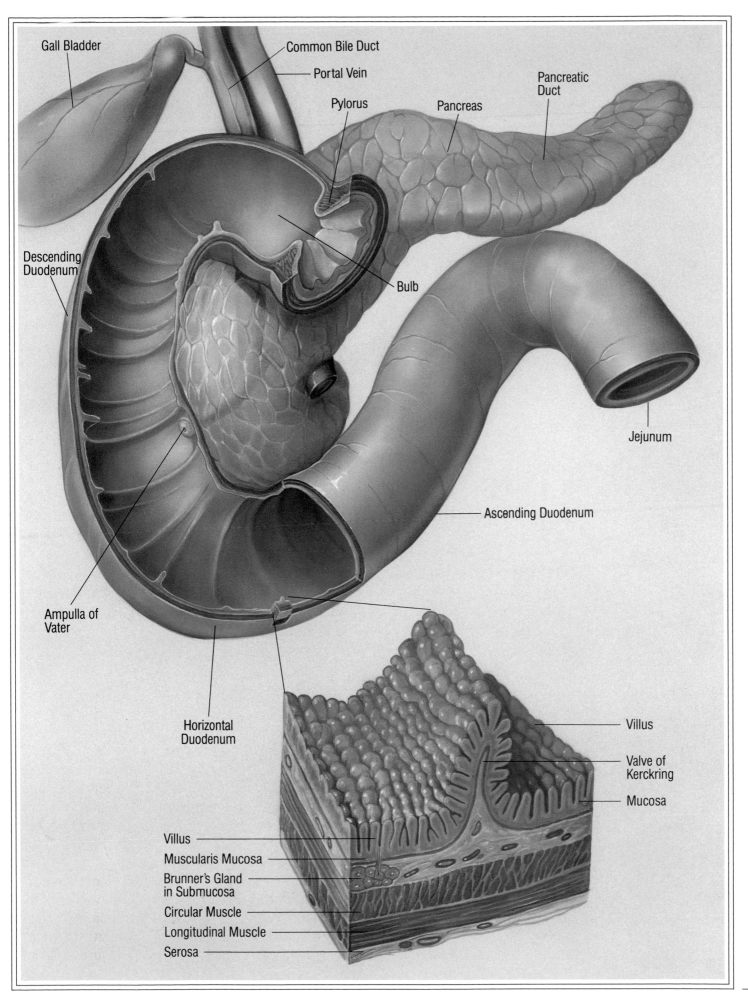

Gall Bladder

Common Bile Duct

Portal Vein

Pylorus

Pancreas

Pancreatic Duct

Descending Duodenum

Bulb

Jejunum

Ampulla of Vater

Ascending Duodenum

Horizontal Duodenum

Villus

Valve of Kerckring

Mucosa

Villus

Muscularis Mucosa

Brunner's Gland in Submucosa

Circular Muscle

Longitudinal Muscle

Serosa

32

Figure 30. Overview of the anatomy of the duodenum.

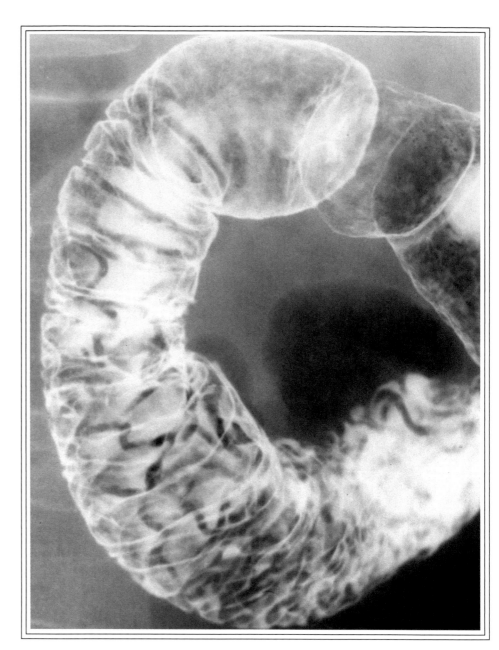

Figure 31. Double contrast radiogram of the duodenum. X-ray provided by I. Laufer.

In the duodenum *in vivo*, a brief exposure to luminal acid results in a sustained rise in bicarbonate secretion. It appears to be dependent on the luminal pH, with a more acidic solution causing a greater increase in bicarbonate secretion. One interesting phenomenon is the rise in duodenal mucosal bicarbonate secretion that occurs simultaneously with gastric secretion of H^+ ions. This simultaneous secretion suggests the existence of an additional mechanism for protection of the duodenum from the effects of acid. There is also a concomitant increase in prostaglandin E_2 release into the luminal perfusate. Both responses are inhibited by pretreatment with indomethacin. They can also be antagonized by specific cholinergic and opiate antagonists such as atropine, hexamethonium, or naloxone, suggesting an involvement of cholinergic and opiate pathways in the neurohormonal control of bicarbonate secretion. VIP may contribute to the control of bicarbonate secretion since VIP-containing cells have been seen in the duodenum. VIP is a potent stimulator of bicarbonate secretion, and luminal acidification results in concomitant secretion of bicarbonate and VIP.

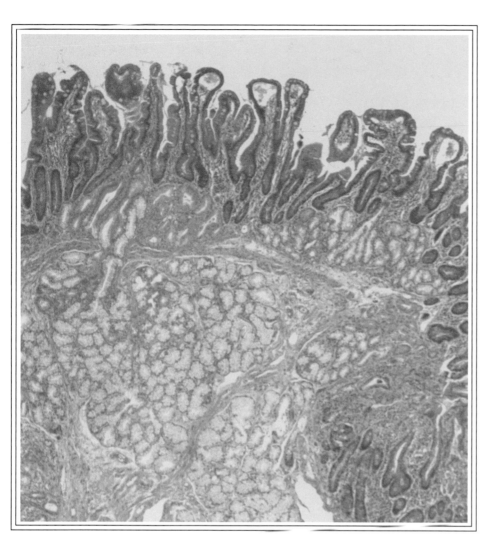

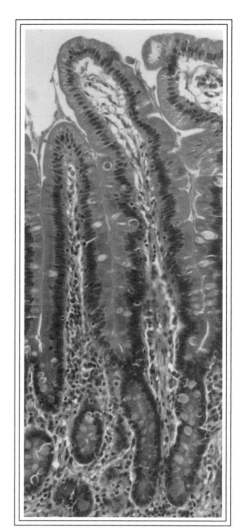

Figure 32. Histology of the duodenal mucosa showing Brunner's glands (left, low power). The villus structure of the epithelium is also shown (right, high power). Micrographs provided by S.H. Saul.

The physiological role of duodenal bicarbonate is unclear, however, since it is difficult to quantitate relative to the pancreatic secretion of bicarbonate, which is thought to contribute to the neutralization of acid discharged from the stomach. It seems likely that secretion of bicarbonate from the duodenum, which enhances mucosal protection by elevating the pH at the epithelial surface, is more important than its effect on the pH in the luminal bulk solution.

Brunner's Glands

Brunner's glands are submucosal, beneath the muscularis mucosa, except in the area close to the pylorus where they may be mucosal. They are located between the pyloro-duodenal junction and the area around the papilla although in younger people they may extend all the way to the jejunum. Histologically, they are seen as branched tubules into which acini open. The ducts drain into the base or side of the mucosal crypts (Figure 33). Two types of cells have been described: mucous (light) and serous (dark) cells. Electron microscopy reveals an elaborate endoplasmic reticulum.

Figure 33. Brunner's glands.

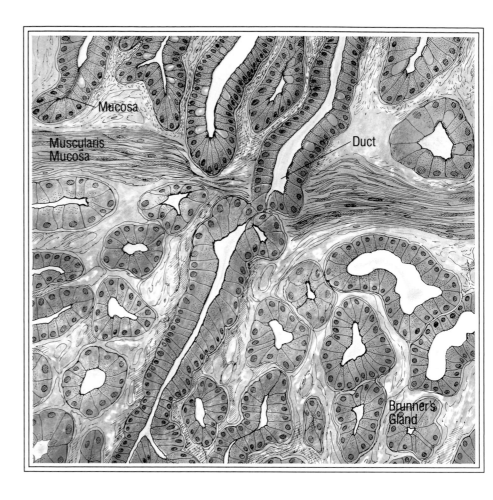

These glands secrete spontaneously and are stimulated by luminal and neurohormonal factors. The finding that secretion of mucous and bicarbonate tends to decrease from the proximal to the distal duodenum suggests that a portion of these secretions comes from Brunner's glands.

Weak acid solutions entering into the duodenum and food, either in the stomach or in the duodenum, can stimulate the secretion of mucous and bicarbonate. As in the duodenal surface epithelium, secretion from Brunner's glands is stimulated by VIP or glucagon and inhibited by aspirin.

1. Grundy D: Gastrointestinal Motility: *The Integration of Physiological Mechanisms.* Lancaster, England, MTP Press Ltd., 1985.

2. Goyal RK and Cobb BW: Motility of the pharynx, esophagus, and esophageal sphincters, in Johnson LR (ed): *Physiology of the Gastrointestinal Tract.* New York, Raven Press, 1981, vol I, chap 11, pp 359-391.

3. Pope II CE: Anatomy and developmental anomalies, in Sleisenger MH, Fordtran JS (eds): Gastrointestinal disease: *Pathophysiology, Diagnosis, and Management, ed 3.* Philadelphia, W.B. Saunders Co, 1983, chaps 24-25, pp 407-422.

4. Spiro HM: *Clinical Gastroenterology, ed 3.* Toronto, McMillan Publishing Co, 1983.

5. Ito S: Functional gastric morphology, in Johnson LR (ed): *Physiology of the Gastrointestinal Tract, ed 2.* New York, Raven Press, 1987, vol 1, chap 26, pp 817-852.

6. Sachs G: The gastric proton pump: The H^+, K^+—ATPase, in Johnson LR (ed): *Physiology of the Gastrointestinal Tract, ed 2.* New York, Raven Press, 1987, vol 1, chap 28, pp 865-882.

7. Debas HT: Peripheral regulation of gastric acid secretion, in Johnson LR (ed): *Physiology of the Gastrointestinal Tract, ed 2.* New York, Raven Press, 1987, vol 2, chap 31, pp 931-946.

8. Hersey SJ: Pepsinogen secretion, in Johnson LR (ed): *Physiology of the Gastrointestinal Tract, ed 2.* New York, Raven Press, 1987, vol 2, chap 32, pp 947-958.

9. Donaldson RM: Intrinsic factor and the transport of cobalamin, in Johnson LR (ed): *Physiology of the Gastrointestinal Tract, ed 2.* New York, Raven Press, 1987, vol 2, chap 33, pp 959-973.

10. Neutra MR, Forstner JF: Gastrointestinal mucus: synthesis, secretion, and function, in Johnson LR (ed): *Physiology of the Gastrointestinal Tract, ed 2.* New York, Raven Press, 1987, vol 2, chap 34, pp 975-1009.

11. Flemstrom G: Gastric and duodenal mucosal bicarbonate secretion, in Johnson LR (ed): *Physiology of the Gastrointestinal Tract, ed 2.* New York, Raven Press, 1987, vol 2, chap 35, pp 1011-1030.

James C. Reynolds, M.D.

PATHOPHYSIOLOGY AND CLINICAL ASPECTS OF
PEPTIC ULCER DISEASE

Introduction

Figure 34. Annual office visits for acid
peptic disease.

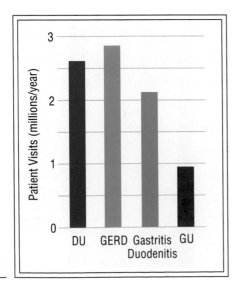

Peptic ulcer diseases afflict millions
of Americans yearly, imposing tremendous personal and financial cost
(Figure 34). Peptic ulcer disease is said to occur sometime in the lives of
4% to 15% of women and 10% to 15% of men in industrialized countries. Not only are these disorders a major cause of abdominal pain, but
the resulting complications may be life threatening. The cost of peptic
ulcer disease in the United States is estimated to be in excess of four
billion dollars per year. This figure includes direct costs, accounting for
40% to 50% of the total costs, and indirect costs, resulting from disability and absenteeism from work. There has been a dramatic increase in
the use of therapies for peptic ulcer disease in the past decade. Over 15
million prescriptions for H_2 antagonists are written on a yearly basis.

While the number of patients receiving treatment for peptic ulcer disease increases yearly, the diagnosis of duodenal ulcer (DU), the most
common form of peptic ulcer disease, has been made less frequently
over the past three decades as our understanding of other types of peptic ulcer disease has increased. During the last decade in particular, the
use of endoscopy has contributed enormously to our understanding of
ulcer disease and expanded its definition. Chronic, penetrating ulcers,
that can be recognized with even the most crude radiographic techniques, have been well described for many years. It has been only
recently understood that the majority of peptic ulcers may actually consist of numerous small erosions (Figure 35). These shallow erosions
rarely lead to perforation but can bleed or progress to a deeper penetrating ulceration. Terms such as esophagitis, gastritis, stress-induced
mucosal disease, and duodenitis are used to describe these more
superficial ulcerating conditions.

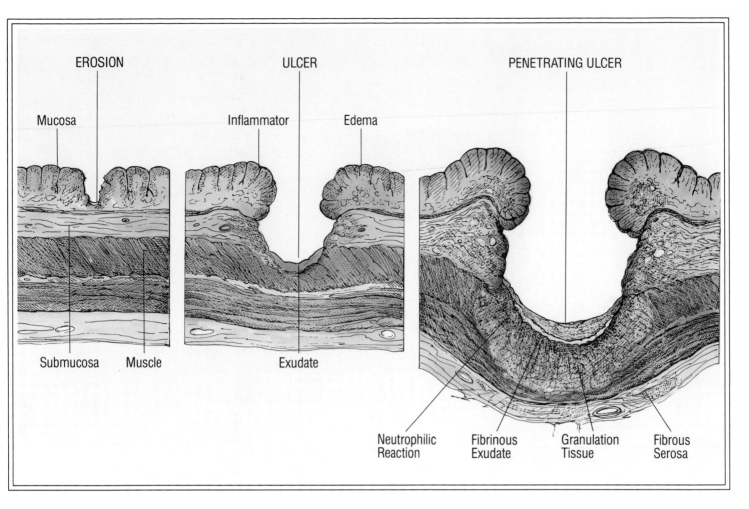

Figure 35. Variable penetration of peptic ulcers.

Endoscopy has also better defined the natural history of ulcerative disorders. It is now known that many ulcer relapses are asymptomatic. For example, while duodenal ulcer was previously thought to be an acute disorder, we now know that a majority of patients with a duodenal ulcer will have a recurrence of the ulcer within 12 months after discontinuation of therapy, regardless of the duration of therapy (Figure 36). Gastric ulcers (GU) are also likely to recur when medications are discontinued. Interestingly, patients who have previously had gastric ulcers tend to have a recurrence of gastric ulcer while those with duodenal ulcers tend to have a recurrence in the duodenum. The chronic nature of peptic ulcer disease must be considered in planning treatment if the frequency of complications is to be reduced.

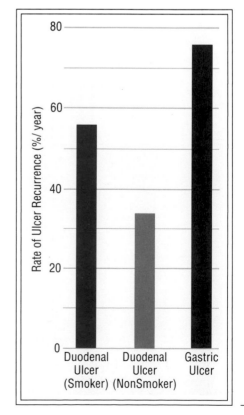

Figure 36. Annual recurrence rate of peptic ulcers after discontinuation of therapy.

Complications of Peptic Ulcer Disease

Complications, including intractable pain, hemorrhage, obstruction, and perforation, and those resulting from ulcer surgery, may affect as many as one fourth of the total number of patients who develop peptic ulcer disease. Sixty percent to 75% of patients with peptic ulcer disease will present with pain as their primary complaint. Pain may vary in intensity from a mild hungerlike discomfort to intractable, excruciating pain. Most interestingly, patients frequently have no pain or the remission of pain early in the course of treatment despite the presence of a large ulcer crater.

Bleeding occurs in 12% to 17% of patients with peptic ulcer diseases. The severity of bleeding varies from mild guaiac-positive stool to chronic iron deficiency anemia to life-threatening arterial hemorrhage. Obstruction may result from chronic fibrosis and scarring of narrow areas of the upper gastrointestinal tract related to recurrent acid-pepsin damage. Strictures occur most commonly in the distal esophagus and pyloric sphincter. Perforation occurs uncommonly but can be the cause of acute abdominal crisis and life-threatening sepsis.

Overview

Peptic ulcer disease results from an imbalance between aggressive and protective factors, specifically, from the corrosive action of acid-pepsin and other intraluminal contents out of balance with mucosal protective factors (Figure 37). Any mucosal surface exposed to gastric contents, a solution of hydrochloric acid and pepsin, can develop mucosal damage, which may progress from erosions to deep ulcerations (Figure 35). Therefore, peptic ulcer disease can affect any of the upper gastrointestinal organs, including the esophagus, stomach, and duodenum. In the presence of a surgically induced gastro-jejunostomy, peptic ulcer disease may occur at the margin of the anastamosis. It is only because of the efficiency of the defensive factors of these organs that peptic ulcer diseases do not occur more commonly in the presence of the very caustic contents of the upper gastrointestinal tract.

Figure 37. Normal balance between aggressive and defensive factors.

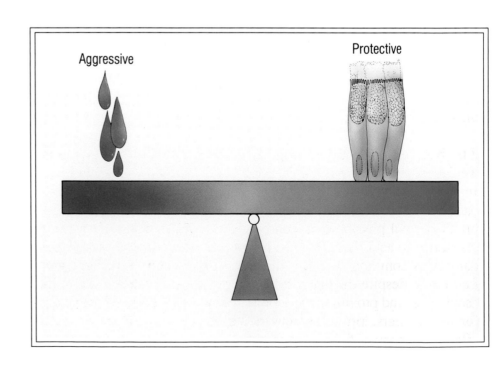

Acid is a necessary factor in the pathogenesis of all forms of peptic ulcer disease, leading to the adage, "No acid, no ulcer." For this reason, most pathophysiological studies of peptic ulcer disease have evaluated the mechanisms of acid secretion and delineated the factors that stimulate the secretion of acid. Clinically, acid secretion is measured by performing a gastric analysis (Figure 38) to quantitate the volume of acid secretion per hour in the basal state and in response to stimulation with the hormone pentagastrin. From such studies it is clear that in patients with duodenal ulcer disease there is an imbalance in the factors regulating the secretion of hydrochloric acid. Furthermore, patients with the most severe and intractable forms of peptic ulcer disease, such as the Zollinger-Ellison syndrome (gastrinoma), also have the highest rates of acid secretion (Figure 39). In contrast, in patients with known achlorhydria (inability to secrete acid), the presence of ulceration by endoscopy or radiography strongly suggests the presence of a malignancy.

Damage to the underlying mucosa in the presence of acid occurs through back-diffusion of hydrogen ions across the mucosal epithelium to underlying structures (Figure 40). Once across the mucosa, the high concentrations of hydrochloric acid present within the stomach cause damage to underlying cellular structures, including neurons, blood vessels, and inflammatory cells. This cellular damage initiates a cascade of secondary events: (1) the release of neurotransmitters that further stimulate acid secretion; (2) the diffusion into the lumen of serum proteins and blood, which are broken down by intraluminal peptidases to amino acids that further stimulate acid secretion; and (3) the activation of intestinal inflammatory cells releasing substances that can act directly to stimulate parietal cell function. Histamine is the most important of the factors released by this inflammatory reaction. Therefore, following the initial diffusion of acid across the mucosal barrier, there is a cascade of events that further promote mucosal damage and acid secretion.

This back-diffusion model, originally proposed by Davenport, has been well accepted as the mechanism of most forms of peptic ulcer disease. In the laboratory, however, it is surprisingly difficult to demonstrate back-diffusion of hydrogen ions across normal mucosa, suggesting that under normal physiological conditions important factors that maintain resistance to acid damage must be present. Furthermore, while peptic damage is common, the fact that it does not occur with even greater frequency, despite the daily and nightly exposure of the stomach, distal esophagus, and proximal duodenum to a very concentrated acid solution for many years, provides convincing circumstantial evidence that effective defensive factors are in place.

Imbalance Between Aggressive and Protective Factors

Figure 38. Gastric analysis. Basal and stimulated secretory outputs are determined by collecting four 15 minute samples before and after stimulation with pentagastrin IV.

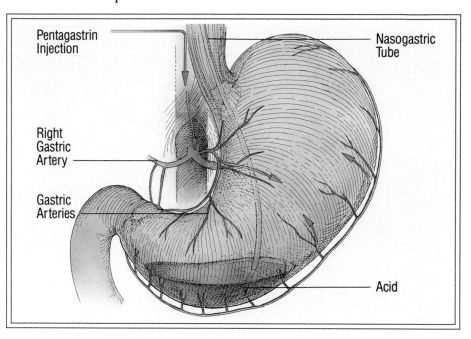

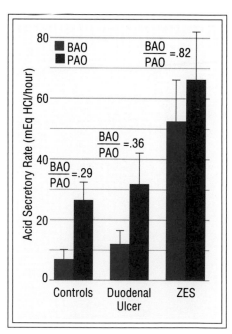

Figure 39. Acid secretory rates. Basal acid output (BAO) and/or peak acid output (PAO) may be increased in patients with duodenal ulcers. In Zollinger-Ellison syndrome (ZES) the ratio of BAO/PAO is >0.6.

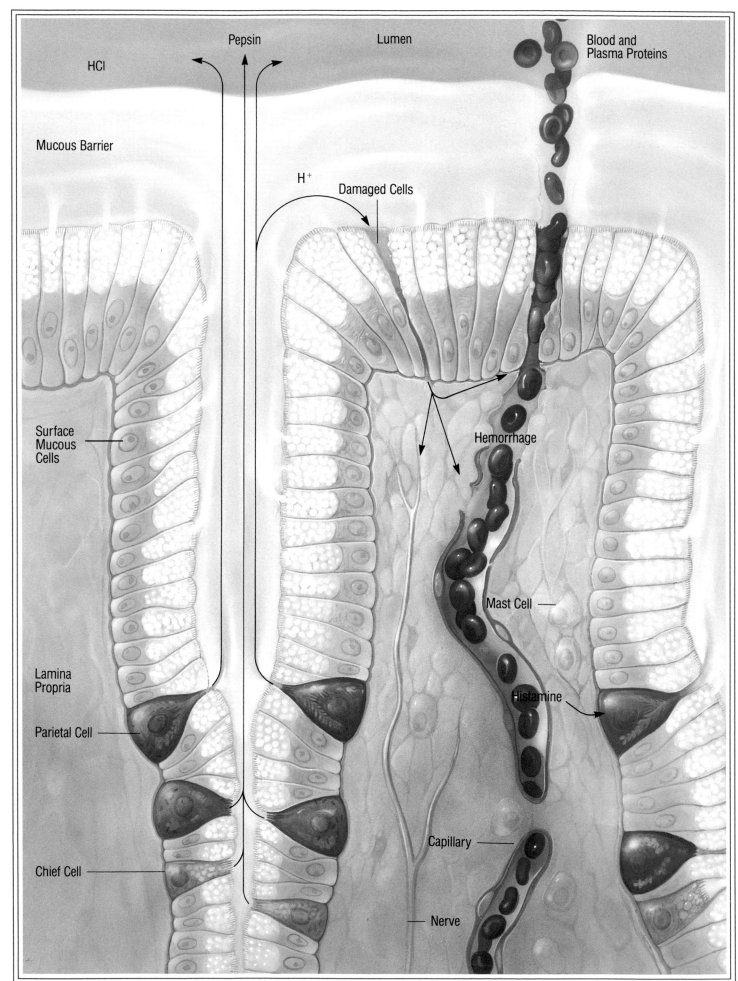

Figure 40. Pathophysiology of peptic ulcer. Adapted from Davenport, *N Engl J Med*, 1967;276:1312.

While acid is the permissive factor leading to peptic ulcer disease, this does not necessarily imply that all patients with peptic ulcer disease secrete excessive amounts of hydrochloric acid (Figure 41). Many patients, even those with duodenal ulcer disease, have basal and peak rates of acid secretion similar to those seen in controls. In several forms of benign gastric ulcer, the peak acid secretory capability of patients is even less than that seen in the normal controls. Increased acid exposure alone is not usually sufficient to cause mucosal damage.

The importance of increased acid secretion as a cause of peptic ulcer disease is perhaps best demonstrated in patients who have a tumor that secretes the hormone gastrin. Zollinger and Ellison were the first to describe these patients as having a syndrome characterized by acid hypersecretion, intractable ulcer disease and pancreatic tumors. Typically, in patients with Zollinger-Ellison syndrome (ZES), as a result of the autonomous secretion of the acid-stimulating hormone gastrin, the rate of acid secretion during fasting (the basal state) is similar to the rate of peak acid secretion in normal subjects (Figure 39). While the rate of acid secretion often reaches dramatic levels, the absolute rate of acid secretion may not be diagnostic. Still, when one compares the rate of basal acid secretion (BAO) with the peak acid secretory rate (PAO) in the vast majority of patients, the ratio will exceed 0.6.

Most patients with Zollinger-Ellison syndrome present with duodenal ulcers, both at the duodenal bulb and distal duodenum. While classically described as recurrent, intractable, large, multiple, or distal ulcerations, the ulcers have no distinguishing features in most patients. Gastric ulcers and esophagitis are less commonly seen in this condition. Diarrhea occurs frequently, as a consequence of damage to the mucosal absorptive surface of the small bowel, the increased volume of secretions, the damage to duodenal regulatory hormone-secreting cells, lipase inactivation, and bile salt precipitation. Elimination of the acid hypersecretory state by resection of the gastrinoma or by pharmacologic intervention also eliminates the predilection to duodenal and gastric ulcerations. Thus, all of the symptoms of the most pernicious ulcer disease are due to acid hypersecretion.

Patients hospitalized with accidental or surgical trauma to the central nervous system also have a high incidence of peptic ulcer disease (Figure 42). The volume of acid secretion over time in patients with trauma to the central nervous system is greatly increased compared with that of control subjects or even subjects who have apparently comparable postoperative stress or pain related to abdominal surgery. This condition was first described by Cushing and bears his name. It is clear that the underlying mechanism of ulcer disease in these patients is a result of an increase in acid secretion that is related to enhanced vagal tone.

Figure 41. Variability of peak acid output in normal controls compared to patients with gastric or duodenal ulcers. Adapted from Wormsley, et al, *Gut,* 1965;6:431.

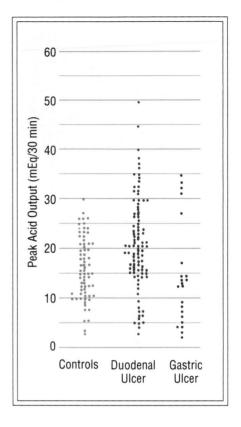

Figure 42. Daily acid secretion in postoperative patients. Adapted from Stremple, et al, *Arch Surg,* 1972;105:179.

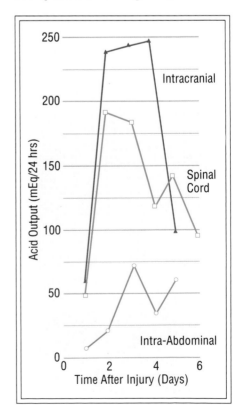

Patients hospitalized with severe burns also have an enhanced risk of developing so-called Curling's ulcers (Figure 43). Despite the clear relationship between the severity of the burn injury and the risk of peptic ulcer disease, these patients secrete less acid than control subjects. Furthermore, there is an inverse relationship between the extent of surface burn and the rate of acid secretion. Thus, while acid is a necessary factor for the development of peptic ulcer disease in burn patients and can be prevented with medications that block acid secretion, mucosal damage is not due to an increased rate of acid secretion. In burn patients under stress, therefore, the primary factor causing ulcer disease appears to be a decrease in mucosal defense factors.

In the most common forms of peptic ulcer disease, including both duodenal ulcers and gastric ulcers, the imbalance between acid hypersecretion and mucosal protective factors is intermediate between these two extremes (Figure 44). In most patients with duodenal ulcers and in those with distal antral (pre-pyloric) gastric ulcers (type II), there is an enhanced secretion of acid and an impaired negative feedback loop to reduce gastrin and acid secretion. In patients with gastric ulcers that occur high in the body of the stomach (type I), the situation is reversed, as these patients secrete less acid than normal, suggesting the importance of impaired mucosal defenses. Furthermore, while the incidence of ulcer disease increases with age, the acid secretory rate decreases in the elderly.

Figure 43. Incidence of Curling's ulcers is a function of the severity of burn. Adapted from Pruitt, et al, *Ann Surg,* 1970;172:529.

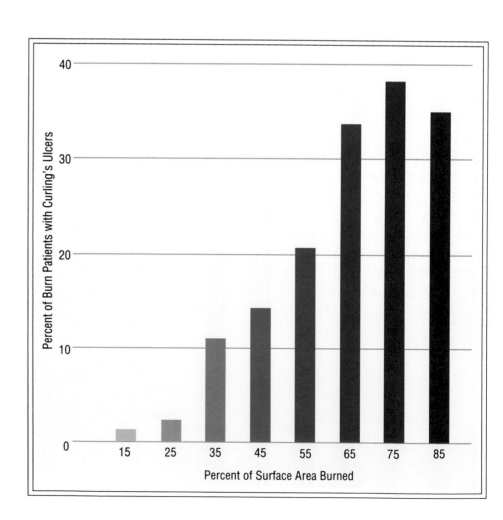

Thus, we can summarize the mechanisms of a given peptic ulcer disease as the result of varying degrees of increased influence of aggressive factors or a decreased presence of protective factors (Figure 44). In conditions such as Zollinger-Ellison syndrome and Cushing's syndrome, acid hypersecretion is a principal pathophysiologic abnormality. In other patients, such as those with a gastric ulcer in the upper part of the stomach or Curling's ulcerations a decrease in the protective factors results in peptic ulcer disease. Acid secretion in a majority of patients lies between these two extremes, and there is an interaction between an increased presence of aggressive factors and a decrease in protective factors.

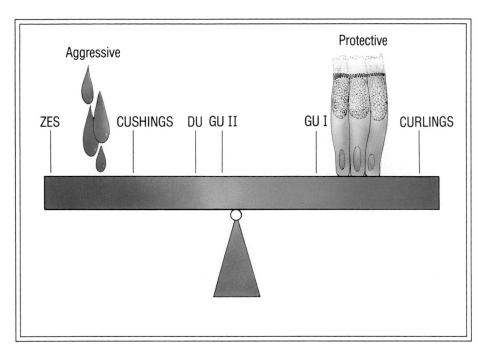

Figure 44. Imbalance between aggressive and protective factors in disease.

Aggressive factors that damage the mucosa of the upper gastrointestinal tract may originate endogenously or may be consumed by a patient (Figure 45). It has been clearly demonstrated that an interaction between these aggressive factors makes the combined effect of multiple "aggressive factors" significantly more caustic to the mucosa than would be seen with the presence of a single factor. This is most clear for pepsin, which is inactive at pH 4 and irreversibly inactivated if the pH is greater than 8. Potentiation of damage results from enhanced hydrogen ion back-diffusion in the presence of bile and pepsin (Figure 40).

Aggressive Factors

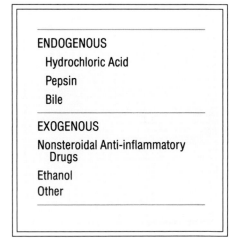

Figure 45. Exogenous and endogenous factors associated with the development of ulcers.

Hydrochloric Acid: The back-diffusion of hydrogen ions is a principal cause of nearly all forms of peptic ulcer disease. It may result from acid hypersecretion, a decreased protection of the tissue from hydrogen ions, or an increased exposure time of duodenal or esophageal mucosa to a low pH. Acid hypersecretion may occur not only in such conditions as Zollinger-Ellison syndrome and duodenal ulcer, as discussed above, but it may also occur at night when there is inadequate intraluminal foodstuff to neutralize acid that is secreted. Nocturnal acid hypersecretion is a particularly important cause of duodenal ulcer disease. Patients with acid hypersecretion generally have an increased sensitivity of parietal cells to secretagogues including histamine and gastrin.

Figure 46. Hypergastrinemic states.

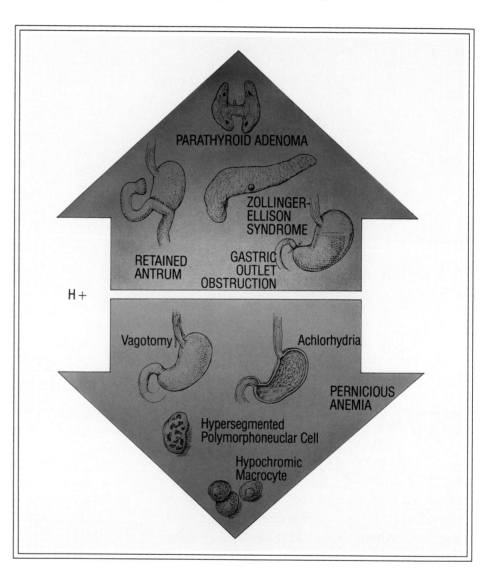

In addition to the Zollinger-Ellison syndrome, other forms of hypergastrinemia are seen (Figure 46). Hypergastrinemic states that lead to peptic ulcer disease are associated with increased hydrogen ion secretion. In other patients, the hypergastrinemia is due to decreased hydrogen ion secretion and release of increased amounts of gastrin occurs in response to alkaline intragastric contents. These conditions include vagotomy, atrophic gastritis, pernicious anemia, and the presence of very potent inhibitors of acid secretion such as H^+/K^+—ATPase inhibitors.

Pepsin: Pepsin, secreted from the chief cells of the antral mucosa, is a potent proteolytic enzyme. In the presence of sufficient hydrochloric acid to activate the conversion of pepsinogen to pepsin, proteolytic activity is enhanced (Figure 47). Pepsinogen is actually a family of proteolytic enzymes of similar structure. In families with increased circulating levels of pepsinogen I, there is an enhanced incidence of peptic ulcer disease. It is possible that certain isomers of the enzyme are more potent in producing proteolysis and mucosal damage. Surprisingly, despite the separate cellular source of pepsin compared with acid, specific syndromes associated with an increase or decrease of pepsinogen secretion have not been reported to cause distinct syndromes of peptic ulcer disease.

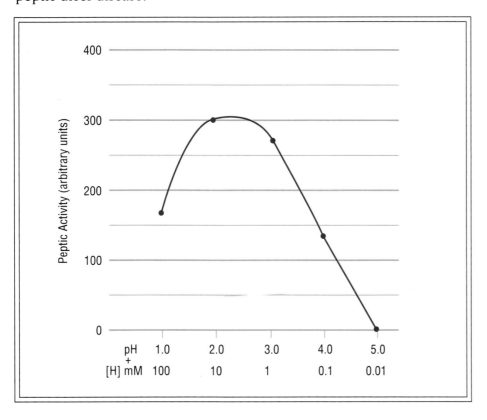

Figure 47. pH dependence of peptic activity.

Bile and Pancreatic Secretions: The potent enzymes and amphipathic bile salts secreted into the duodenum can have a caustic effect on gastric and esophageal mucosa. In the presence of motility disorders or surgical derangement of the normal anatomy, bile refluxes into the stomach or esophagus where mucosal damage often occurs. Bile acids, primarily lithocholic acid, are thought to be the most caustic components in bile, and they frequently cause mucosal damage. There is little question, however, that other proteolytic enzymes and lipases contribute to this effect. Reflux of bile has been reported to cause not only diffuse mucosal damage but, in rare instances, the complications of peptic ulcer disease of the esophagus, including Barrett's metaplasia. Despite the importance of bile and pancreatic enzymes in producing ulcers, inhibition of acid secretion often results in healing, suggesting that hydrogen ions are still important in most patients who have bile reflux gastritis.

Exogenous Mucosal Irritants

Studies of the role of diet in the pathophysiology of duodenal and gastric ulcers have implicated a surprisingly small list of agents associated with ulcerogenesis (Figure 48). While a large number of therapeutic agents are irritating to the stomach, they rarely lead to frank ulceration. Agents in this group include multivalent cations (such as iron and calcium), antibiotics (such as erythromycin and tetracycline), and cardiovascular medications (such as reserpine and quinidine).

Alcohol: Ethanol has a predictable, concentration-dependent, damaging effect on the mucosa of the esophagus and stomach. An acute inflammatory and hemorrhagic lesion will be induced in the vast majority of healthy individuals by the rapid ingestion of ethanol. Alcohol is a contributing factor in over one third of patients presenting with acute upper gastrointestinal hemorrhage. High concentrations of alcohol cause denuding of the superficial mucosal cells extending to the midfundic glands, resulting in intramucosal hemorrhage, increased permeability, and, to a lesser extent, an inflammatory infiltrate.

Aspirin and Nonsteroidal Anti-Inflammatory Agents (NSAIDs): Endoscopic studies indicate that gastric erosions will develop in virtually anyone who ingests therapeutic doses of aspirin on a regular basis. Intravenous administration of salicylates has no significant effect on mucosal permeability or on epithelial integrity as examined by light or electron microscopy. Both aspirin and nonsteroidal anti-inflammatory agents inhibit the synthesis of prostaglandins, which have an important role in normal mucosal defense. Mucous secretion is also reduced. Acid enhances the damage induced by increasing the absorption of aspirin, since unionized aspirin in the presence of a low pH is absorbed better than is the ionized form of the molecule. Epithelial permeability, as measured by a decrease in the electrical potential difference (PD) across the mucosa from lumen to serosa, is decreased in a concentration-dependent fashion by aspirin, perhaps by inhibition of the chloride pump (Figure 49). The increase in permeability due to ingestion of aspirin is further increased by coadministration of alcohol. There is also a reduction in mucous and bicarbonate secretion. Tight junctions (Figure 50), however, remain intact. Both aspirin and pepsin will potentiate the damaging effect of alcohol on the gastric epithelium.

Smoking: Smoking has an unequivocally adverse effect on the epithelium of the upper gastrointestinal tract, which significantly increases the prevalence of acid peptic damage. In smokers the risk of developing a duodenal ulcer is increased fivefold over that for nonsmokers. Smoking also significantly reduces the probability of spontaneous ulcer healing and perhaps the rate of healing in response to treatment.

Figure 48. Risk factors for peptic ulcer disease.

RISK FACTORS FOR PEPTIC ULCER DISEASE

Coffee

Alcohol

Tobacco

Salicylates

Heredity

NSAIDS

Age

Figure 49. Effect of aspirin (ASA) on epithelial permeability. Adapted from Murray, et al, *Br Med J,* 1974;1:19-20.

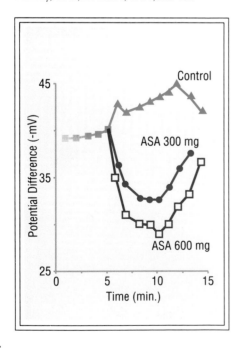

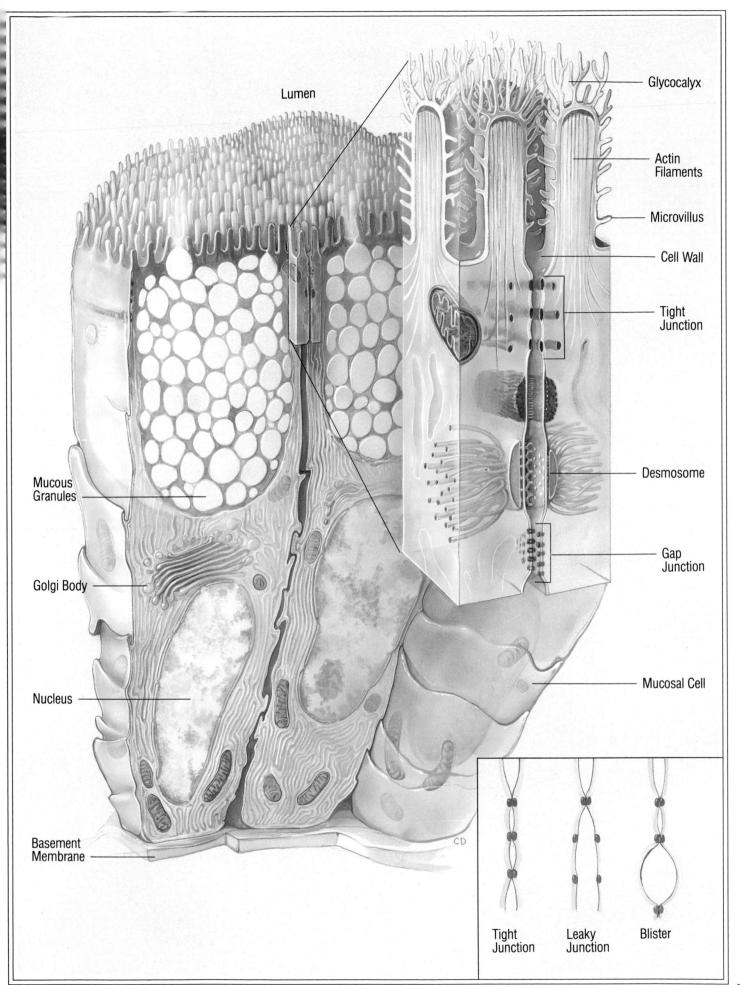

Lumen

Glycocalyx

Actin Filaments

Microvillus

Cell Wall

Tight Junction

Desmosome

Gap Junction

Mucosal Cell

Mucous Granules

Golgi Body

Nucleus

Basement Membrane

Tight Junction

Leaky Junction

Blister

48

Figure 50. Junctional organelles of gastric mucosal epithelium. Adapted from Powell, *Am J Physiol*, 1981;241:6275-6288.

The most convincing evidence implicating smoking in the development of duodenal ulcers is that the incidence of ulcer recurrence in patients who continue to smoke is almost twice the incidence in non-smokers or in patients who discontinue smoking (Figure 36). Smoking reduces the pH of intraduodenal contents, probably by decreasing bicarbonate secretion (Figure 51).

Coffee and Caffeine: Caffeine acts synergistically with histamine (but not pentagastrin) to stimulate acid secretion. It also enhances the secretion of pepsin. Interestingly, both regular coffee and decaffeinated coffee are more potent stimuli of acid and pepsin secretion than is caffeine alone, suggesting that a constituent of coffee, in addition to caffeine, has a significant effect on gastric secretion.

Abnormalities of Protective Factors

After examining the caustic nature of intraluminal contents, it is surprising that the incidence of peptic ulcer disease is not greater. The tremendous efficiency and high rate of synthesis of protective factors prevent a greater incidence of peptic ulcer disease from occurring. These protective factors include mucous secretion (Figure 52), bicarbonate synthesis, and prostaglandin secretion (Figure 53). The integrity of the mucosal barrier is also enhanced by a rapid rate of cell turnover and mucosal blood flow.

Mucous: Mucin is a complex polymer of glycoproteins (Figure 52). An increased rate of depolymerization of mucous has been shown to be an important factor in the etiology of gastric ulcers. Experimentally, mucous degradation reduces the normal transmucosal pH gradient (Figure 40). Pepsin and other proteolytic enzymes are able to degrade normally depolymerized mucous molecules thus decreasing their ability to impair the diffusion of hydrogen ions (Figure 52).

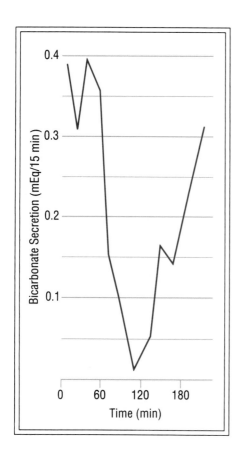

Figure 51. Smoking impairs pancreatic bicarbonate secretion. Adapted from Murthy, et al, *Gastroenterology*, 1977; 73:759.

Figure 52. Glycoprotein polymers of mucin are subject to proteolysis. Figure modified from Clamp, et al, *Br Med Bull*, 1978;34:31.

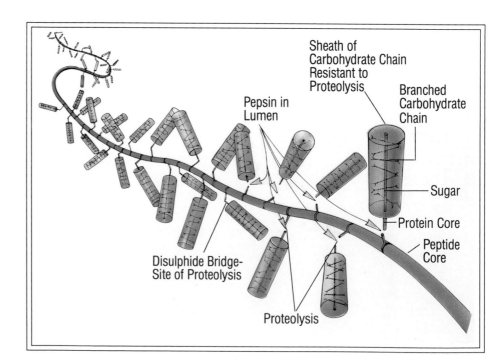

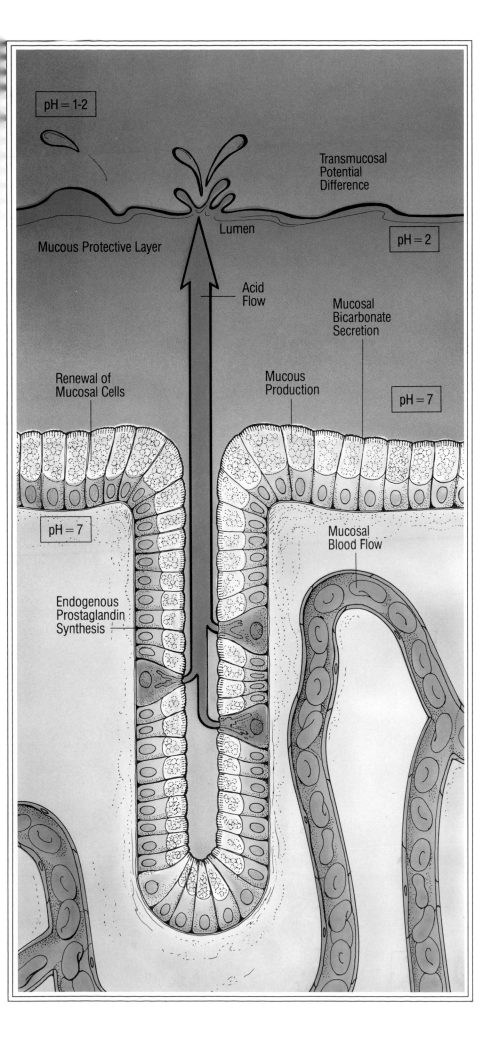

pH = 1-2

Transmucosal
Potential
Difference

Lumen

Mucous Protective Layer

pH = 2

Acid
Flow

Mucosal
Bicarbonate
Secretion

Renewal of
Mucosal Cells

Mucous
Production

pH = 7

pH = 7

Mucosal
Blood Flow

Endogenous
Prostaglandin
Synthesis

Figure 53. Mucosal protective factors.

50

Bicarbonate: Mucosal bicarbonate secretion also contributes to the defense of the lining of the stomach and duodenum. Acid within the lumen of the duodenum is neutralized by bicarbonate secreted from the pancreas. Convincing evidence that decreased bicarbonate is important in the pathogenesis of duodenal ulcer disease comes from studies of patients who are heavy smokers and have a decreased pancreatic bicarbonate secretory capacity (Figure 51). It has been suggested that bicarbonate secretion from the oral mucosa may also be important in the prevention of esophagitis.

Blood Flow: The high metabolic rate of the gastric and duodenal epithelium requires a high blood flow to maintain oxygenation and nutrition. In shock and other low flow conditions, mesenteric blood flow is shunted to the systemic circulation to maintain perfusion. This peripheral shunting is often accomplished at the expense of adequate flow to the mucosa. Such shunting is a major factor in the etiology of stress-related mucosal disease and acute hemorrhagic gastritis. Shunting of mesenteric blood flow to the periphery has also been proposed as an explanation of the gastric mucosal damage seen in marathon runners.

Figure 54. Reepithelialization of damaged mucosa.

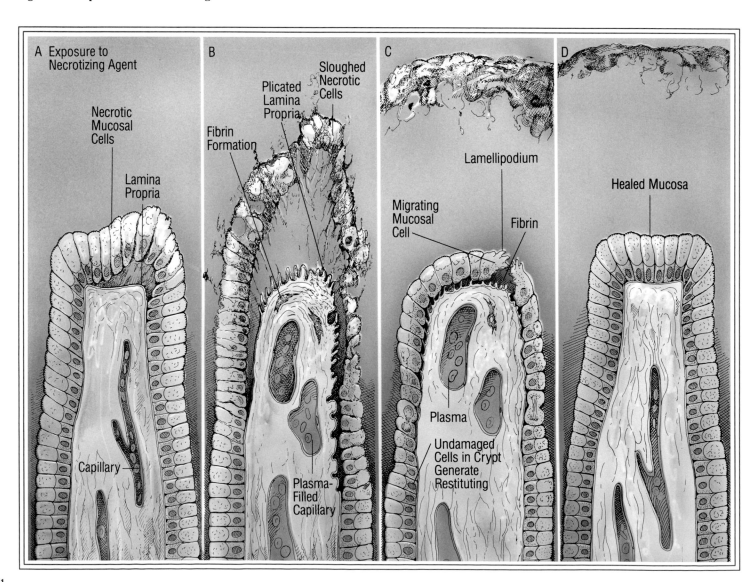

Mucosal Cell Turnover: The epithelium of the stomach is renewed every third day, a rate exceeded only by the bone marrow. Such turnover is particularly important in the presence of the caustic gastric contents, which are constantly attacking the more mature cells at the tips of the glands (Figure 54). Re-epithelialization is an important normal process in protecting the mucosa from the intermittent damage associated with the ingestion of gastric irritants such as alcohol and aspirin (Figure 54). In the presence of irritants, the normal cytoskeletal matrix on which the epithelium rests becomes denuded. Cell migration and rapid cell turnover quickly repairs the injury.

DUODENAL ULCER

The importance of duodenal ulcer disease is manifested by its prevalence, its potential for life-threatening complications, and its cost to society. Duodenal ulcers are the single most common cause of hemodynamically significant upper intestinal bleeding. Duodenal ulcer disease may affect up to 10% of the male population of the United States. Perhaps as a consequence of these observations, no peptic ulcer disease has been studied as extensively as have duodenal ulcers.

Specific Pathophysiologic Mechanisms in Duodenal Ulcer Disease

Several physiologic abnormalities have been shown to be present in many, but not all, patients with duodenal ulcer disease (Figure 55). The common causative factor in these abnormalities is an increased delivery of insufficiently buffered hydrochloric acid to the duodenum (Figure 56). An increase in acid secretion both in the basal state and in response to stimulants has been described in patients with duodenal ulcers. Basal acid secretion is variable, but is most consistently elevated at night. This nocturnal hypersecretion of acid in duodenal ulcers has important therapeutic implications. Maximal acid secretion is variable, even among duodenal ulcer subjects, as discussed previously (Figure 41). When duodenal ulcer patients are compared with controls, there is a significant increase in acid secretion in the ulcer patient group. The presence of increased acid secretion in both the cephalic phase (sham feeding and insulin hypoglycemia) and gastric phase (gastric distention) of acid secretion suggests that an increased parietal cell mass is present in many patients.

Acid secretion in response to a meal can be calculated by analysis of titratable acidity within the stomach or in aspirated specimens. Acid secretion in response to a meal has been shown to be increased in some patients with duodenal ulcers.

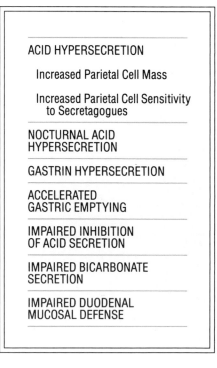

ACID HYPERSECRETION

Increased Parietal Cell Mass

Increased Parietal Cell Sensitivity to Secretagogues

NOCTURNAL ACID HYPERSECRETION

GASTRIN HYPERSECRETION

ACCELERATED GASTRIC EMPTYING

IMPAIRED INHIBITION OF ACID SECRETION

IMPAIRED BICARBONATE SECRETION

IMPAIRED DUODENAL MUCOSAL DEFENSE

Figure 55. Physiologic abnormalities in patients with duodenal ulcers.

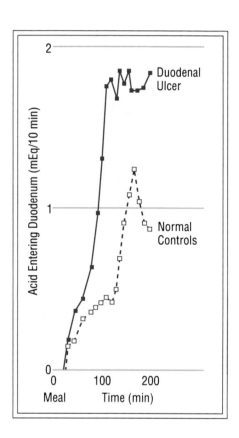

Figure 56. Acid delivered to the duodenum is increased in subjects with ulcers. Adapted from Malagelada, et al, *Gastroenterology,* 1977;73:989-994.

Following a meal, patients with duodenal ulcers demonstrate an abnormally rapid delivery of acid to the duodenum and a prolonged increase in acid secretion as compared with normal subjects (Figure 56). The prolonged acid hypersecretion suggests that the increased acid delivery to the duodenum results not only from an increased capacity to secrete acid, but also from an inability of duodenal receptors in these patients to feed back a sufficient inhibitory response to the gastric secretory mucosa. Studies of the feedback inhibitory pathways influencing acid secretion, however, have resulted in variable findings with regard to the importance of impaired inhibitory factors. The inhibitory effects of secretin, cholecystokinin, somatostatin, glucagon, and several test meals in duodenal ulcer subjects is similar to that seen in controls.

Several lines of evidence suggest that there is also hypersecretion of pepsinogen in some patients with duodenal ulcer. These patients have increased circulating levels of pepsinogen, increased levels of pepsinogen in gastric secretions, and an increased rate of pepsin secretion that parallels hypersecretion of acid.

Hypersecretion of acid and pepsin may be due in part to the increased activity of gastrin in patients with duodenal ulcer disease. The peak level and time integrated serum concentration of gastrin is elevated in these patients even in the absence of gastrinoma or gastric surgery. In light of the frequency of acid hypersecretion in duodenal ulcer, this tendency toward gastrin hypersecretion is significant, suggesting that feedback inhibitory systems are impaired. The inhibition of gastrin secretion in response to somatostatin is less in ulcer patients than in controls.

The importance of altered mucosal defense mechanisms in duodenal ulcer patients is controversial. Despite the consistent finding of an overall increase in mean acid secretory capacity in groups of duodenal ulcer patients, the acid secretory rate of nearly two thirds of individual subjects will be within normal limits (Figure 41). In up to 40% of ulcer patients, spontaneous healing can be demonstrated. These factors suggest that mucosal protective factors are important, even in patients with active duodenal ulcers. Duodenal secretion of bicarbonate is an important aspect of duodenal mucosal defense. Proximal duodenal bicarbonate secretion per unit of surface area is nearly five times greater than in gastric mucosa and nearly twice that seen in the distal duodenum. Experimental models of duodenal ulcer disease induced in the rat with cysteamine or mepirizole are associated with reduced secretion of alkali. The concentration of the duodenal mucosal prostaglandin 6-keto-PGF is actually increased in patients with duodenal ulcers, as is the luminal secretion of PGE. Both of these prostanoids have cytoprotective effects, and their secretion may be altered as a response to ulceration. Data implying the importance of other cytoprotective factors in the causation of duodenal ulcer are less convincing although this may be due, at least in part, to the difficulty in adequately assessing these factors.

Motility factors, particularly an enhanced rate of emptying of liquids, have been suggested to play an important role in the development of duodenal ulcers. In several studies the rate of acid delivery to the duodenum has been shown to be enhanced, although the results from other studies suggest that the importance of motility in the development of ulcers is not well resolved. Pyloric sphincter pressures are similar in duodenal ulcer subjects and controls.

In summary, the pathophysiology of duodenal ulcers is complex and multifactorial. No one abnormality can be demonstrated to be responsible for the development of mucosal damage in all patients, suggesting that heterogeneous mechanisms are present. Acid and pepsinogen hypersecretion and increased delivery to the duodenum can be demonstrated to be present in the majority of patients and, thus, appear to be the most important factors in the development of an ulcer.

Risk Factors for Developing a Duodenal Ulcer

The suspicion of duodenal ulcer should be heightened in the presence of a family history of duodenal ulcer, smoking, or excess caffeine use. Of the gastric irritants discussed above (Figure 48), smoking and caffeine use have been most clearly associated with an increased risk of developing a duodenal ulcer. Smoking increases the risk of developing an ulcer and the likelihood of ulcer recurrence, while it reduces the likelihood of spontaneous healing. Some studies have shown that smoking has no effect on the rate of ulcer healing, but this observation remains controversial. The rate of ulcer recurrence is nearly doubled in patients who smoke cigarettes on a daily basis. Of all risk factors, smoking has the greatest influence on the incidence and recurrence of duodenal ulcer. Acid and pepsin hypersecretion that occur in response to caffeine and coffee increase the incidence of duodenal ulcers in patients who ingest these substances. The ingestion of corticosteroids may increase the incidence of duodenal ulcerations. The data is less convincing that alcohol, aspirin, and nonsteroidal anti-inflammatory drugs affect the likelihood of developing a duodenal ulcer.

Analysis of genetic factors through twin and blood group studies is consistent with a genetic predisposition to the development of duodenal ulcers. There is a threefold increased risk of developing a duodenal ulcer in first degree relatives of patients with duodenal ulcers. The incidence of duodenal ulcer in males exceeds that in females by 2:1. A family history of ulcer disease not only increases the risk of developing some form of peptic ulcer disease, but a history of duodenal ulcers specifically increases the risk of duodenal ulcers, not gastric ulcers.

Of the hereditary factors that have been shown to influence the incidence of duodenal ulcer disease, the association is the strongest for patients with an increased serum concentration of pepsinogen I (Figure 57). An elevated serum concentration of pepsinogen I is inherited as an autosomal dominant trait. In studies of large families with the trait, duodenal ulcers occurred in half of those with the trait and in none without the trait. Overall, family members with the trait are five times as likely to have a duodenal ulcer as those without it. The development of duodenal ulcers in these patients cannot be solely ascribed to abnormalities in pepsinogen secretion, as the presence of elevated serum levels of pepsinogen appears to be a marker of patients with acid hypersecretion, increased sensitivity to gastrin, postprandial hypergastrinemia, and impaired feedback inhibition of acid secretion.

Figure 57. Autosomal dominant inheritance of pepsinogen I hypersecretion. Adapted from Rotter, et al, *N Engl J Med,* 1979; 300:63-66.

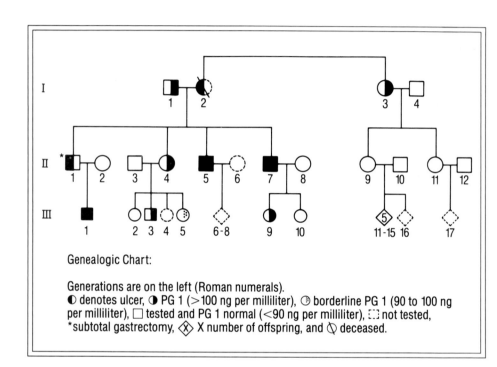

Other markers of hereditary predisposition have been identified, but the association is less secure than with hereditary pepsinogenemia. Patients with duodenal ulcers have an increased frequency of blood Group O. They are also more likely to be found not to secrete blood group antigens ABH into their saliva.

Clinical Presentation

Duodenal ulcers classically present with epigastric to right upper quadrant pain. This pain may radiate to either side of the epigastrum, or may mimic the pain of pancreatitis by radiating posteriorly, particularly in the presence of a posterior penetrating ulcer. The pain is often most intense 2 to 4 hours after eating and often awakens the patient from sleep. The pain is typically reduced by the ingestion of milk, food, or antacids. In other patients the pain may be vague, diffuse, and without relationship to eating. Although pain is the hallmark symptom in ulcer disease, it is an unreliable indicator of the presence or absence of ulcer healing.

While the presence of an ulcer may be predicted by the presence of a typical symptom complex, up to 25% of patients have no pain prior to the development of significant complications of a duodenal ulcer, including upper intestinal bleeding. Bleeding may be manifested by vomiting of fresh blood (hematemesis) or digested blood (coffee ground emesis), or by the passage of black, tarry stools (melena). Less commonly, the patient will develop an iron deficiency anemia due to chronic, recurrent bleeding. The severity of bleeding depends on the size of the blood vessel involved and will vary from melena to a life-threatening loss of blood. Duodenal ulcers may also present with symptoms of other complications such as penetration, perforation, or obstruction, as described below.

Less commonly, patients with a duodenal ulcer may present with vague, nonspecific complaints often referred to as dyspeptic symptoms. These include bloating, anorexia, nausea, and unexplained vomiting. Patients presenting with nonspecific complaints such as bloating, "gas," belching or unexplained weight loss may be difficult to diagnose until an ulcer is detected by X-ray or endoscopy.

Before pursuing the diagnosis of duodenal ulcer with upper gastrointestinal radiographs or endoscopy, a careful physical examination should be performed with particular attention to details that suggest the presence of complications. The blood pressure and pulse should be examined in the supine and upright postures, particularly when bleeding is suspected. Tenderness in the right upper quadrant or epigastrum is a frequent physical finding. The presence of decreased bowel sounds, particularly when associated with signs of peritonitis such as guarding or rebound, suggests the possibility of a penetrating or perforating ulcer. Hyperactive bowel sounds are often present in patients with upper gastrointestinal bleeding because of the cathartic effect of blood. The possibility of bleeding should be evaluated in all patients by examining the stool for occult or gross blood, and, when appropriate, by passing a nasogastric tube and lavaging the stomach as the patient attempts to induce reflux of duodenal contents by performing a Valsalva maneuver. A nasogastric tube is also a valuable means of evaluating the patient for impaired gastric emptying, particularly when a succussion splash is detected by physical examination.

Diagnosis of Duodenal Ulceration

The specific diagnosis of a duodenal ulcer can be made by visualization of the ulcer through radiographic (Figure 58) or endoscopic techniques (Figure 59). The vast majority of duodenal ulcers will occur within the first three centimeters of the pylorus, in the duodenal bulb (or cap). In the presence of ulceration, the normal smooth contour of this triangularly shaped region is replaced by an ulcer crater or mucosal erosion. A rim of edema may give the impression of a mass extending into the lumen. Often the radiologist will report that there is evidence of peptic ulcer disease without being able to demonstrate a specific ulcer crater. Radiographic findings that suggest peptic ulcer disease involving the duodenum include deformity, thickened folds, eccentricity of the pyloric orifice, and spasm. A giant duodenal ulceration with smooth contours may resemble a large duodenal bulb and thus be difficult to detect radiographically.

Deformity or spasms of the bulb may mask the ulcer crater. The use of double contrast techniques can reduce the incidence of false-negative studies and help to determine whether mucosal deformity represents ulceration, scar, or edema. Abdominal compression, prone views, and oblique views will also increase the sensitivity of this noninvasive technique.

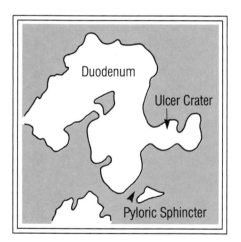

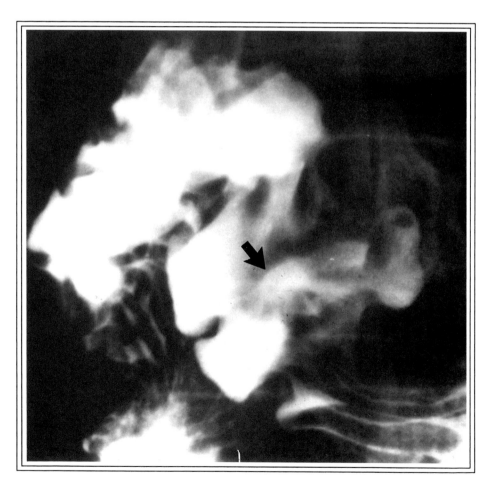

Figure 58. Radiographic appearance of duodenal ulcer. Radiograph provided by I. Laufer.

Fiberoptic or video endoscopic techniques allow for direct visualization and the unequivocal diagnosis of duodenal ulceration (Figure 59). The normal, pale pink color of the mucosa is replaced by a yellow crater that is often surrounded by a rim of erythema. The surrounding mucosa often shows less severe evidence of acid peptic damage with edema, erythema, and friability. Submucosal nodules, commonly seen in the first and second portions of the duodenum, represent reactive hyperplasia of Brunner's glands. Endoscopy typically requires mild sedation and anesthetization of the pharyngeal mucosa but is both a specific and a highly sensitive diagnostic tool.

Ulcerations may be round or oval in shape and can be seen in any part of the bulb or in the pyloric channel between the duodenum and antrum. Multiple ulcerations will be seen in 15% to 20% of patients. The presence of multiple post-bulbar ulcerations should raise the clinical suspicion of Zollinger-Ellison syndrome (gastrinoma). Ulcer size is variable and correlates poorly with the severity of symptoms. The majority of ulcers are less than 1 cm in diameter, and 15% will be less than 4 mm. Endoscopy may also detect the presence of superficial erosions and diffuse mucosal edema throughout the proximal duodenum leading to the diagnosis of duodenitis.

The hallmark of duodenal ulcer is denudation of the normal mucosal epithelium (Figure 60A,B). The eroded epithelium will be replaced with a fibrinous exudate and polymorphonuclear cellular infiltrate. The depth of penetration will vary from superficial erosions to deep chronic ulcers that begin to penetrate into adjacent structures. Adjacent mucosa will show villus blunting with separation of glandular elements by an inflammatory infiltrate. Brunner's glands are often hyperplastic, with glandular elements extending both above and below the muscularis mucosa.

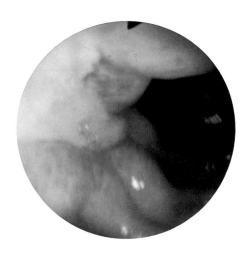

Figure 59. Endoscopic appearance of duodenal ulcer. Endoscopy provided by J.C. Reynolds.

Pathologic Features of Duodenal Ulcers

Figure 60A and B. Gross and microscopic pathology of duodenal ulcer. Photographs provided by S.H. Saul.

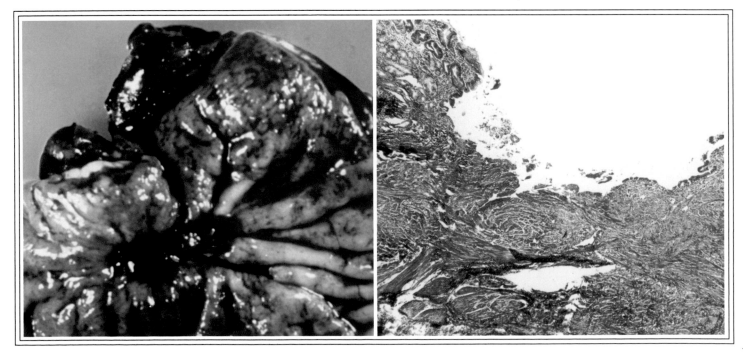

Complications of Duodenal Ulcer
Disease

Bleeding: Gastrointestinal bleeding occurs in 20% of patients with duodenal ulcer. Bleeding is responsible for over half of the deaths associated with duodenal ulcer disease and is the most common reason for emergent surgical treatment of active duodenal ulcers. The severity of duodenal ulcer bleeding varies from occult blood in the stool, to the development of iron deficiency anemia, to a life-threatening acute bleed. While the hospital mortality associated with a duodenal ulcer bleed is less than 5% in young, otherwise healthy patients, it is much higher in subjects with massive or recurrent bleeds or those with other serious medical problems. Ulcer healing is significantly impaired in patients with a history of duodenal ulcer bleeding. Such patients should receive at least 8 weeks of intensive medical therapy to assure healing.

A bleeding duodenal ulcer should be suspected when the patient presents with symptoms of melena or hematemesis or when examination of the stool by guaiac testing is positive. Nasogastric aspiration of the stomach will determine whether the bleeding is active. The patient should be asked to perform a Valsalva manuever to induce the reflux of duodenal contents into the stomach before suggesting that a duodenal ulcer is not bleeding. Only the direct visualization of the ulcer by endoscopy can definitively determine whether active bleeding is present or not (Figure 61).

Several endoscopic findings have been associated with recurrence or persistence of duodenal ulcer bleeding. These findings include prolonged or recurrent bleeding on therapy, a visible vessel, or a large adherent clot over the ulcer. Such patients should receive surgical consultation, and endoscopic interventional therapy should be considered.

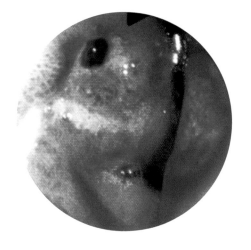

Figure 61. Visible vessel in a previously bleeding duodenal ulcer. Endoscopy provided by E. Morgan.

Obstruction: Early satiety, vomiting of foodstuff hours after a meal, or the physical finding of a succussion splash suggests the presence of gastric outlet obstruction (Figure 62A). This complication occurs in 1% to 5% of patients with a duodenal ulcer. Despite the overall decrease in the incidence of uncomplicated duodenal ulcers and the dramatic decrease in elective surgery for this condition in the past two decades, the frequency of hospital admissions for gastric outlet obstruction has not decreased. Endoscopic or radiographic evaluation will demonstrate an enlarged gastric cavity with stenosis of the pyloric channel or distal duodenal bulb. Because of the chronic nature of this complication, an active ulcer is an inconsistent finding. In many patients, pyloric stenosis can be corrected by endoscopically directed pneumatic dilatation with balloons of increasing diameter followed by prolonged, intense medical therapy. In others, surgery is unavoidable if adequate nutrition is to be obtained.

Penetration and Perforation: Penetration and perforation occur in less than 1% of all duodenal ulcers. Penetration most often occurs into adjacent organs of the gastrointestinal tract, including the pancreas, stomach (double outlet sign), or the biliary tract (Figure 62B). Penetration into the biliary tract most commonly occurs between the posterior duodenal bulb and the underlying common bile duct. Air in the biliary tract is the hallmark radiographic finding on plain abdominal X-ray. Interestingly, such patients typically have excellent results with medical therapy alone.

Penetration into the pleural space, pericardium, and liver have been reported less frequently. Penetration of a duodenal ulcer into the aorta has been reported most commonly in patients who have had a previous abdominal aortic aneurism repair. In this circumstance the presence of the aorto-duodenal fistula in the distal duodenum suggests that graft infection, recurrent aneurism, or local trauma has contributed to the usual causes of duodenal ulcers in developing this life-threatening complication. The patient typically presents with abdominal pain and a brisk upper intestinal bleeding that heralds a subsequent exsanguinating bleed. Fever and other signs of infection are inconsistent findings. Prompt diagnostic evaluation and surgical intervention are essential.

Free perforation of a duodenal ulcer, which occurs uncommonly, may produce life-threatening peritonitis and is a surgical emergency (Figure 62C). Less commonly, subphrenic air can be found during roentgenographic examination of a patient who presents with less acute symptoms. In the absence of findings suggesting peritonitis, these patients can be cautiously treated with medical therapy alone.

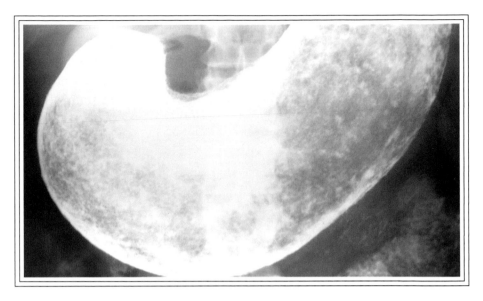

Figure 62A. Obstruction. Gastric outlet obstruction has resulted from chronic duodenal ulcer disease and stenosis of the outlet. Radiograph provided by I. Laufer.

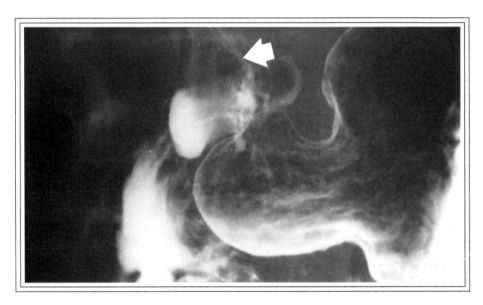

Figure 62B. Choledochoduodenal fistula. Orally injected contrast fills the common bile duct through an ulcer-induced fistulous tract (arrow). Radiograph provided by I. Laufer.

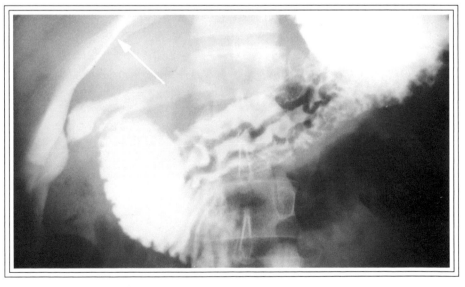

Figure 62C. Free perforation. Contrast has collected beneath the liver (arrow). Radiograph provided by I. Laufer.

GASTRIC ULCER

The incidence of gastric ulcers has increased in a linear fashion over the past four decades. Gastric ulcers tend to occur in patients who are 10 to 15 years older than the average patient with a duodenal ulcer. Thus, as the mean age of our population increases, it is likely that the incidence of gastric ulcers will also continue to increase. While the pathophysiologic mechanisms and clinical features of gastric ulcers in the distal antrum are similar to those of duodenal ulcers, several lines of evidence suggest that ulcers occurring in the midbody and corpus have several distinctive features. The discussion of gastric ulcers that follows specifically refers to this subset of patients with gastric ulcer. Patients with stress-induced gastric mucosal damage are discussed in the next section.

The peak age of onset of gastric ulcers is between 60 and 70 years of age. Patients with gastric ulcers have a high incidence of concurrent medical problems. Death occurs more commonly in patients with gastric than duodenal ulcer, but is rarely due to the ulcer disease. The ingestion of other medications is frequently implicated in the development of gastric ulcer disease. As with duodenal ulcer disease, there is a high rate of recurrence of gastric ulcer that has variably been reported to be between 60% and 75%.

Specific Pathophysiologic Mechanisms in Gastric Ulcer Disease

Genetic Factors: There is again a two- to threefold increased risk of developing a gastric ulcer in individuals with first degree relatives with gastric ulcers. As with duodenal ulcers, the site of ulcer formation tends to remain consistent among family members, so that patients with gastric ulcers have an increased risk of developing gastric, but not duodenal, ulcers. In contrast to duodenal ulcers, the male predominance is less pronounced in gastric ulcer patients, best estimates being a 3:2 ratio of males to females.

Acid Secretory Rates: In contrast to the increased rates of secretion of acid and pepsin seen in patients with duodenal and prepyloric ulcers, patients who develop gastric ulcers in the body or fundic mucosa may have low peak acid secretory capacity (Figure 41). In fact, basal acid secretion, nocturnal secretion, titratable acid secretion in response to meal, and maximal acid output as determined by histamine stimulation are all lower in patients with ulcers above the angularis compared with these rates of secretion in healthy controls. Similarly, there is a decreased density of gastrin-secreting cells in the antrum of patients undergoing antrectomy for gastric ulcer when compared with controls and a reduced circulating gastrin level.

Exogenous Aggressive Factors: Aspirin, nonsteroidal anti-inflammatory drugs, and other medications are commonly implicated as causes of gastric ulcers. Salicylates typically induce multiple, superficial ulcerations in the distal stomach along the greater curvature (Figure 63). Aspirin ingestion is associated with an increased risk of upper gastrointestinal bleeding, predominantly from gastric lesions. Bleeding that occurs from such lesions is typically chronic and low volume, although massive bleeding from deep ulcers is not uncommon. While the experimental administration of salicylates intravenously can induce antral ulcers, the incidence of endoscopically documented ulcers is lower in patients who take enteric-coated products. As discussed previously, the damage from salicylates and NSAIDs is most likely due to inhibition of prostaglandin synthesis and increased mucosal permeability.

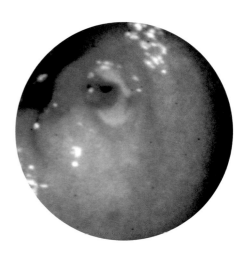

Duodenogastric Reflux: The importance of abnormal gastroduodenal motility in the development of gastric ulcers also distinguishes gastric from duodenal ulcers. A number of investigators have shown that the gastric concentration of bile salts in the basal state and after a meal is increased in patients with gastric but not duodenal ulcers. Pyloric sphincter pressures are lower, and the pyloric contractile response to duodenal acidification is impaired in patients with gastric but not duodenal ulcers. Thus, gastric ulcers may be the result of the reflux of duodenal contents onto an atrophic gastric mucosa with impaired acid secretory capacity. The specific agent responsible for mucosal damage is not known, although most studies implicate bile salts. Bile salt conjugates have been shown to have the capacity to disrupt the mucosal barrier. It is possible that alkali or lysolecithin are contributing factors. Thus, motility abnormalities are an important contributory factor in many patients with gastric ulcers in that they permit the retrograde movement of duodenal contents, primarily bile salts.

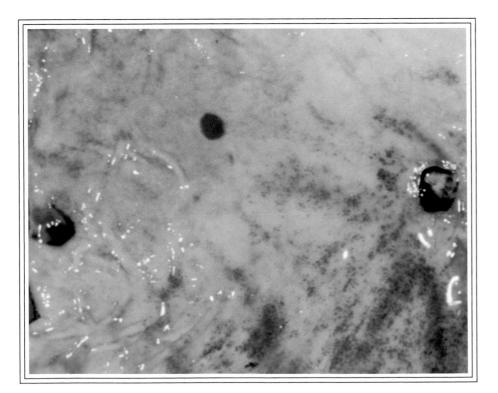

Figure 63. Histologic (left) and endoscopic (above) views of superficial ulcerations caused by ingestion of salicylates. Endoscopy provided by J.C. Reynolds and histologic photograph by S.H. Saul.

Helicobacter pylori: There is evidence that mucosal damage of the upper gastrointestinal tract, primarily the gastric antrum, is associated with the presence of a recently described flagellated bacteria, *Helicobacter pylori*. Histologic staining, cultures, or tests for urea-splitting organisms in the mucosa will confirm the presence of this bacteria in the majority of patients with antritis and in many patients with both duodenal ulcer and antritis (Figure 64). The incidence of recurrent disease is increased in patients from whom this organism can be cultured. Because it is primarily a saphrophyte, with little cytolytic capability, debate continues with regard to the importance of the organism in causing disease of the gastric or duodenal epithelium. Alternatively, it may be a nonspecific marker of cell death and mucosal destruction.

Clinical Presentation of Gastric Ulcers

The clinical presentation of gastric ulcers is frequently indistinguishable from that of gastric malignancy. Ulcers of the proximal antrum, corpus, and fundus tend to occur in the elderly and to present with chronic, recurrent pain. Pain persists for an average of 6 to 8 months in most patients before they seek medical attention. The occurrence of the pain is not predictable but often worsens with eating, resulting in anorexia, sitophobia and weight loss. While weight loss is typically associated with malignant ulcers, 30% to 50% of patients with benign gastric ulcers also experience it. Often the pain radiates to the back. Not uncommonly, the patient's symptoms are vague and can be confused with cardiac or pulmonary disorders. Bleeding occurs in 25% of patients, but gastric obstruction is distinctly uncommon. In contrast to duodenal ulcers, gastric ulcers are clinically, and sometimes radiographically, indistinguishable from adenocarcinoma of the stomach. The presence of a malignancy must be carefully excluded by a thorough radiographic and endoscopic evaluation.

Radiographic and Endoscopic Findings: Both benign (Figure 65) and malignant (Figure 66) gastric ulcers occur most commonly on the lesser curvature of the stomach. While earlier reports suggested that ulcers on the greater curvature were more commonly malignant than benign, this observation has been subsequently refuted. Either benign or malignant ulcers may vary in diameter from a few millimeters to several centimeters. The presence of multiple ulcers favors a benign diagnosis, particularly if a duodenal ulcer is also noted.

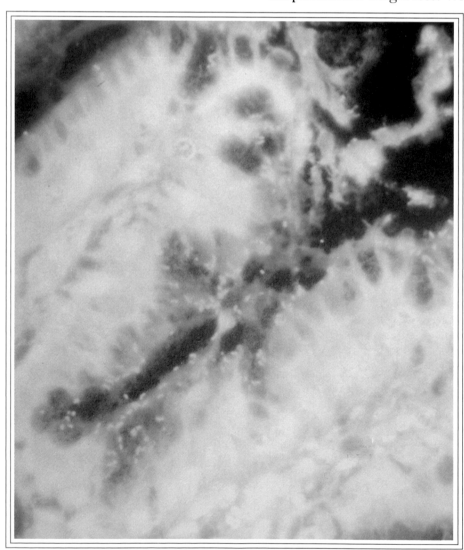

Figure 64. Helicobacter pylori organisms fluoresce above gastric epithelial cells (acridine orange stain, courtesy S. Saul).

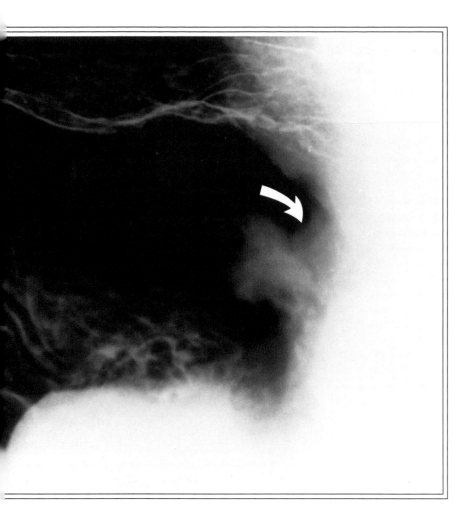

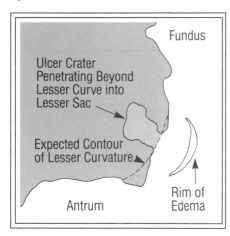

Figure 65. Radiographic appearance of benign gastric ulcer. Radiograph provided by I. Laufer.

Fundus

Ulcer Crater Penetrating Beyond Lesser Curve into Lesser Sac

Expected Contour of Lesser Curvature

Rim of Edema

Antrum

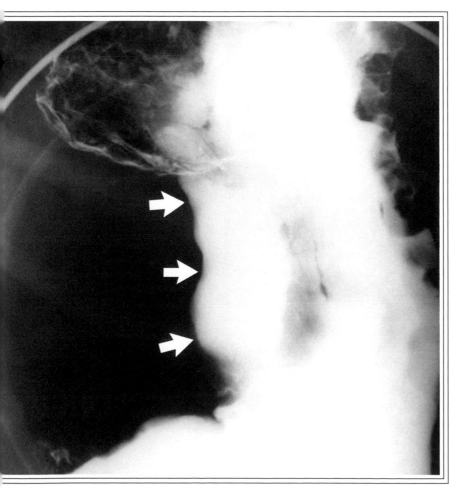

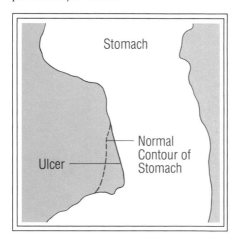

Figure 66. Radiographic appearance of malignant gastric ulcer. Radiograph provided by I. Laufer.

Stomach

Normal Contour of Stomach

Ulcer

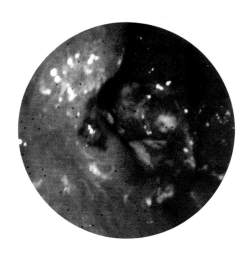

Figure 67. Endoscopic appearance of benign gastric ulcer. Endoscopy provided by J.C. Reynolds.

A number of radiographic features have been identified that help to differentiate benign ulcers from malignant lesions. Complete healing is the most reliable radiographic sign that an ulcer is benign. To accept this sign, however, without tissue confirmation, the lesion must be totally healed. Benign ulcers typically project beyond the contour of the stomach, have radiating folds to the edge of the ulcer, have intact surrounding mucosa, a Hampton line (line of radiolucency representing edema at the base of the ulcer), and an absence of filling defects. Localized rigidity suggests carcinoma. In large series, however, approximately 10% of gastric carcinomas were missed on an initial barium study and 15% of benign ulcers were misdiagnosed as malignant.

Endoscopic biopsies and brushing are the most accurate methods of determining whether a lesion is benign (Figure 67) or malignant. Rigidity, poor distensibility, a mass effect, and interruption of the contour of the surrounding gastric rugae suggest the presence of a malignant lesion. If careful brushings and multiple biopsies are taken, the accuracy of endoscopic evaluation approaches 95%. Most endoscopists would, nevertheless, follow up negative pathologic studies with a second procedure (either endoscopy or X-ray) to make sure that all malignancies are identified.

Pathologic Findings

The characteristic pathologic findings of benign gastric ulcers are illustrated in Figures 68A and 68B. The malignant ulcer shown in Figures 68C and 68D demonstrates how malignant ulcers can mimic benign lesions. The definitive diagnosis of a benign condition clearly requires endoscopic evaluation with biopsies and cytologic analysis.

STRESS-RELATED MUCOSAL DISEASE

Of the common acid peptic diseases, none has a greater risk of leading to severe morbidity or mortality than does stress-related mucosal disease (SRMD). These lesions are characterized by the presence of superficial hemorrhage and ulcerations involving the gastric mucosa of patients with multisystem disease, shock, or sepsis. In contrast to other peptic ulcer diseases, pain occurs uncommonly, and most patients present with signs of bleeding. Clinically apparent bleeding occurs in 20% of patients, while hemodynamically significant bleeds are seen in 5% to 7% of patients. Once a more serious level of bleeding develops, the mortality rate exceeds 50%.

Figure 68A-D (opposite page). Pathologic characteristics of gastric ulcers. The gross appearance of benign gastric ulcer (68A) may be indistinguishable from malignant ulcers (68C). The lack of mass effect, radiation of folds up to the ulcer margin and lack of distortion in Figure 68A strongly support a diagnosis of benign disorder. Penetrating benign ulcers (Figure 68B) produce underlying fibrosis, infiltrates and edema. The signet ring structures in Figure 68D produce a distinctive pattern in this form of gastric malignancy. Photographs provided by S.H. Saul.

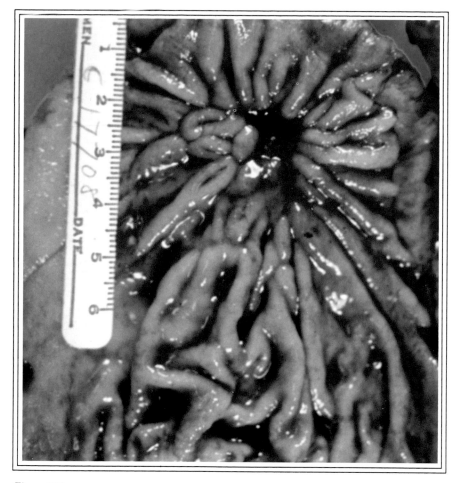

Figure 68A.

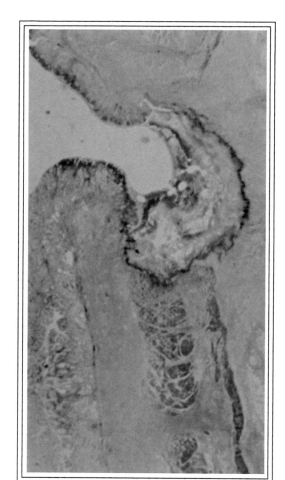

Figure 68B.

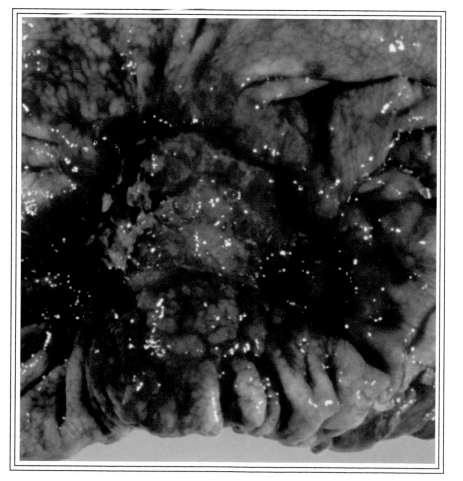

Figure 68C.

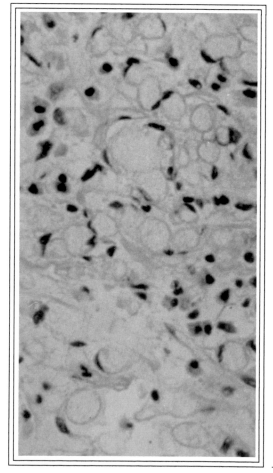

Figure 68D.

66

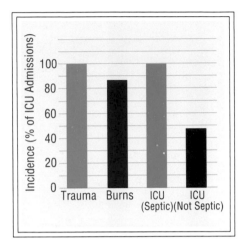

Figure 69. Incidence of stress-related mucosal damage.

The importance of gastric mucosal injury in patients who are under stress because of serious injuries, central nervous system trauma, or burns has been recognized for years, as described in the beginning of this chapter for Cushing's and Curling's ulcers. A small subset of patients were reported from autopsy series and intensive care units to develop massive gastrointestinal bleeding, known as acute hemorrhagic gastritis. Only with the development of endoscopic techniques that could be brought to the patient's bedside to evaluate the cause of minor degrees of bleeding in seriously ill patients could the frequency of this lesion be appreciated (Figure 69). Nearly 100% of patients following central nervous system surgery or trauma, 75% to 85% of general surgery patients, and 60% of patients admitted to medical intensive care units can be shown to have the typical endoscopic findings of stress-related mucosal disease. The incidence of SRMD parallels the severity of the underlying disease (Figure 70).

Several features distinguish the mucosal lesions in patients under extremes of physiologic stress from those who have the more typical chronic peptic ulcer disease. These lesions occur in a setting of trauma, shock, burn, sepsis, and multiple organ failure in patients with no previ-

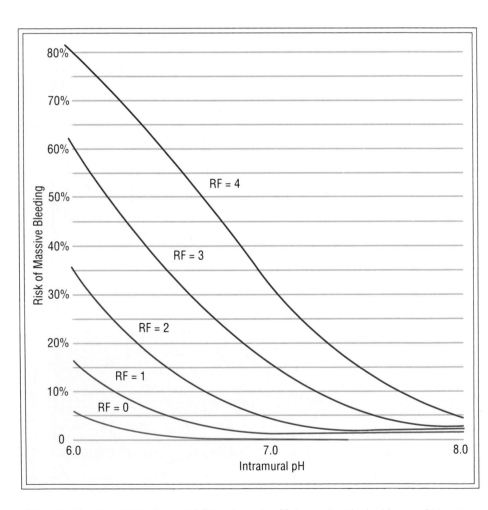

Figure 70. Number of risk factors (RF) and gastric pH determine the incidence of bleeding. Adapted from Fiddian-Green, et al, *Gastroenterology*, 1983;85:617.

ous history of ulcer disease. Stress lesions tend to be multiple (Figure 71) in contrast to the one or two lesions typically found in patients with duodenal or gastric ulcers. SRMD is a diffuse mucosal abnormality that occurs throughout the stomach, although there is a predominance in the acid-secreting mucosa (Figure 72A). In contrast, typical peptic ulcers occur in the nonacid secreting mucosa, the gastric antrum, and the duodenum. SRMD is a superficial mucosal lesion involving the upper half of the gastric glands (Figure 72B) in contrast to typical peptic ulcers that can penetrate through the intestinal wall. Perforations are distinctly uncommon in SRMD but occur in 1% to 2% of patients with gastric and duodenal ulcers. When bleeding occurs in SRMD, therefore, only the venous capillaries are involved in contrast to the larger vessels involved with other peptic ulcers.

The overall outcome in patients with stress-related mucosal disease is dependent primarily on the outcome of their underlying disease. Once the acute catastrophe has cleared, the mucosal injury repairs itself without sequellae. In contrast to typical gastric or duodenal ulcers, there is no tendency toward recurrence, in the absence of recurrence of the underlying disease.

Clinical Presentation

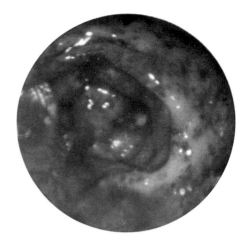

Figure 71. Endoscopic appearance of stress-related muocosal disease. Endoscopy provided by E. Morgan.

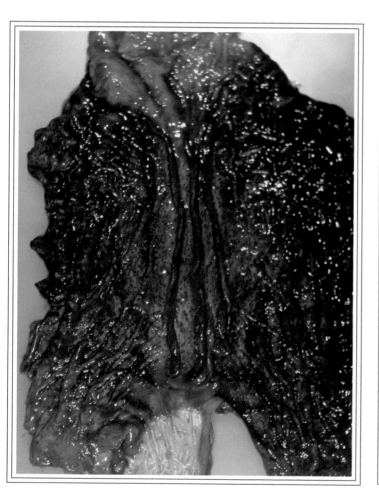

Figure 72A. Diffuse punctate areas of erythema in the acid secretory mucosa of the stomach typify the gross appearance of SRMD.

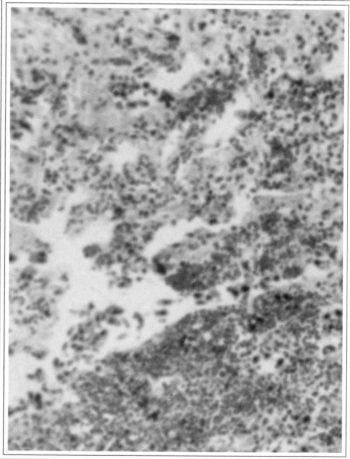

Figure 72B. Histologic appearance of SRMD: sloughing of mucosa and inflammatory cells over a diffuse distribution. Photographs provided by S.H. Saul.

68

Specific Pathophysiologic Mechanisms of Stress-Related Mucosal Disease

The specific mechanisms involved in the development of stress-related mucosal disease are incompletely understood, but most likely involve multifactorial impairment of mucosal defense systems. Key to the initiation of this lesion is the reduction in mesenteric blood flow that accompanies systemic hypotension and shock. The decrease in gastric blood flow results in localized anoxia and ischemic changes. This in turn reduces the ability of the gastric epithelium to undergo the active metabolic processes necessary for mucous and bicarbonate synthesis, cell turnover, and the maintenance of mucosal ionic pumps needed to maintain mucosal integrity.

Endoscopic and Histologic Features

Due to the nature of the patient's underlying disease, radiographic evaluation is seldom possible. Endoscopy can be performed safely in the vast majority of patients at the bedside. The typical, diffuse superficial ulcerations that characterize SRMD are shown in Figures 71 and 72A. The histologic counterpart of this superficial lesion is shown in Figure 72B. Lesions are characterized by intramucosal hermorrhage throughout a wide distribution of the stomach but with little penetration to the deeper submucosa or muscularis propria.

Although it is both common and potentially lethal, SRMD can be prevented by the prompt institution of appropriate antiulcer therapy.

GASTROESOPHAGEAL REFLUX DISEASE

Figure 73. Symptoms of gastroesophageal reflux disease.

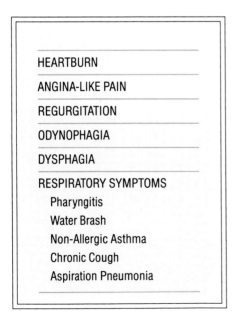

HEARTBURN
ANGINA-LIKE PAIN
REGURGITATION
ODYNOPHAGIA
DYSPHAGIA
RESPIRATORY SYMPTOMS
Pharyngitis
Water Brash
Non-Allergic Asthma
Chronic Cough
Aspiration Pneumonia

Acid-peptic damage to the esophagus results in a variety of clinical symptoms known collectively as gastroesophageal reflux disease (GERD). The symptoms that result from gastroesophageal reflux are listed in Figure 73. The most frequent symptom is heartburn, which is one of the most common gastrointestinal complaints. It has been estimated that 30% of the population of the United States experiences heartburn at least once per month, and some 10% to 15% experience it daily. Twenty-five percent of women in their third trimester of pregnancy will have significant difficulty with heartburn and regurgitation. This very common disorder also has the potential for producing significant morbidity and, in rare cases, even mortality. It is the only peptic ulcer disease known to have the potential to induce a premalignant condition. In the presence of chronic recurrent ulcerative esophagitis, patients may develop a metaplastic change in which the squamous epithelium is converted to columnar epithelium. Barrett's metaplasia is a precancerous lesion, and up to 5% to 10% of patients who develop this condition will develop an adenocarcinoma. Other esophageal complications of chronic reflux esophagitis include bleeding, iron deficiency anemia, and strictures. It has been estimated that 15% to 20% of all patients thought to have severe ischemic heart disease for which they undergo cardiac catheterization are later proven to have normal coronary arteries, with half of these having an esophageal origin of the chest pain. Of these patients, the majority will have gastroesophageal reflux, with or without esophageal spasm. Thus, reflux of the acidic contents of the stomach into the esophagus is a serious cause of not only esophageal disease but of chest pain that can mimic cardiac disease.

Gastroesophageal reflux of acid and other gastric contents not only leads to esophageal problems but has been shown to be an important cause of pulmonary disease. Chronic gastroesophageal reflux can lead to recurrent aspiration and interstitial pneumonitis. Reflux of gastric contents is also an important cause of nosocomial pneumonia in patients who are achlorhydric. Although in the past this disease was seen primarily in the elderly, it is now thought to be a major cause of nosocomial pneumonia in intensive care unit patients in whom stomach acid has been neutralized to prevent stress-related mucosal disease. Thus, patients with gastroesophageal reflux disease may present to physicians with complaints that appear to originate from the pulmonary system, the cardiovascular system, or the abdomen, or they may present with a clear-cut history of reflux esophagitis.

Pathologic degrees of acid reflux result from a variety of mechanisms (Figure 74). The distal esophagus is the only place in the body where the contents of the thoracic cavity, under negative atmospheric pressure, are exposed to the contents of the abdominal cavity, which are under positive pressure. It is only through the maintenance of a high pressure zone at the junction of the esophagus and stomach that acid does not continuously reflux up from the stomach into the esophagus. For acid reflux to occur, therefore, there must be a breakdown in the maintenance of this barrier, the lower esophageal sphincter (LES). Several mechanisms for the breakdown in the maintenance of the lower eosphageal sphincter pressure have been proposed (Figure 75). In patients with serious esophageal reflux disease, including those with the complications of acid reflux, the lower esophageal sphincter is invariably hypotonic throughout much of the day. Therefore the contents of the abdominal cavity under positive pressure exceed the pressure gradient and are able to freely reflux into the esophagus. This is particularly likely when the patient lies flat or increases his intra-abdominal pressure through a Valsalva maneuver, the wearing of tight clothing, or obesity. Fatty foods, progesterone, caffeine, anticholinergic medications, and neuro-muscular disorders can also reduce lower esophageal sphincter pressure (Figure 74).

Mechanisms of Gastroesophageal Reflux Disease

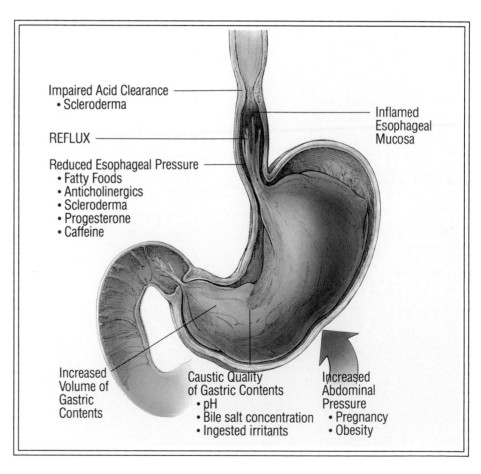

Figure 74. Mechanisms of gastroesophageal reflux.

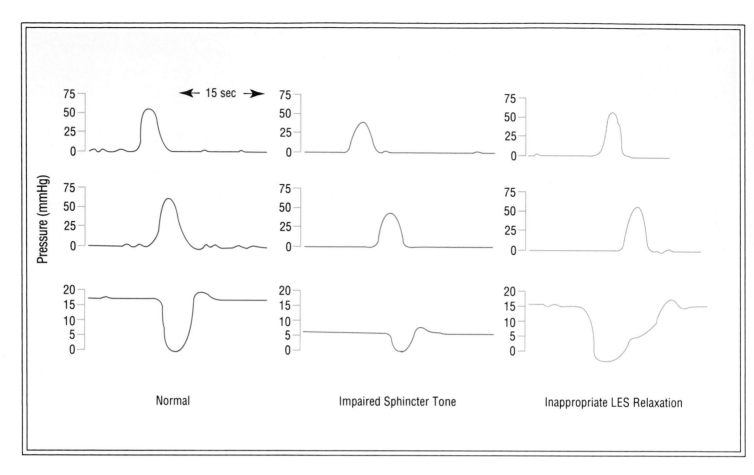

Pressure (mmHg)

← 15 sec →

Normal

Impaired Sphincter Tone

Inappropriate LES Relaxation

Figure 75. Mechanisms of lower esophageal sphincter impairment. The most severe forms of gastroesophageal reflux occur when the normal tonic pressure gradient is replaced by a continuously impaired barrier mechanism. Alternatively LES pressure may be normal for most of the day and relax inappropriately, allowing intermittent acid reflux. Pressure tracing correspond to 10 cm above (top), 5 cm above (middle), and at the LES (lower).

In addition, acid may reflux into the esophagus when a lower esophageal sphincter at normal pressure undergoes intermittent relaxation. This occurs under normal physiologic circumstances during swallowing, particularly in the postprandial period, and during belching in an effort to relieve the increased pressure associated with swallowed air. Thus, the lower esophageal sphincter relaxes intermittently after a meal and with belching, and during these times acid reflux is apt to occur.

It has recently been suggested that intermittent, inappropriate relaxations of the lower esophageal sphincter may occur in the absence of any other identifiable stimulant. According to this hypothesis, inappropriate lower esophageal sphincter relaxation permits acid to reflux into the esophagus. Acid refluxed into the esophagus stimulates a secondary peristaltic contraction and eventual clearance of the acid through peristalsis and the secretion of saliva.

While the presence of an incompetent lower esophageal sphincter, whether on a persistent basis or occurring intermittently, is a necessary requirement for acid reflux, it is not alone sufficient. Through the development of increasingly sophisticated 24-hour intraesophageal pH recordings it has been established that acid refluxes into the esophagus in all normal subjects (Figure 76). This presumably occurs due to normal relaxation of the lower esophageal sphincter associated with inhibitory hormones released in response to meals, gastric distention, or belching.

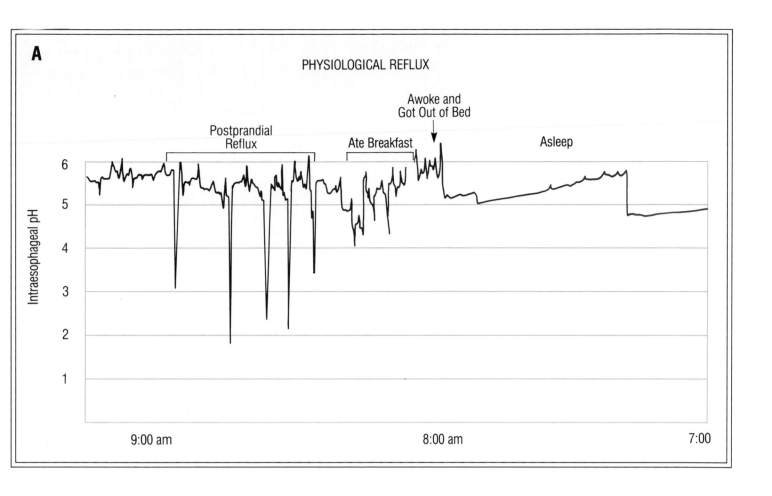

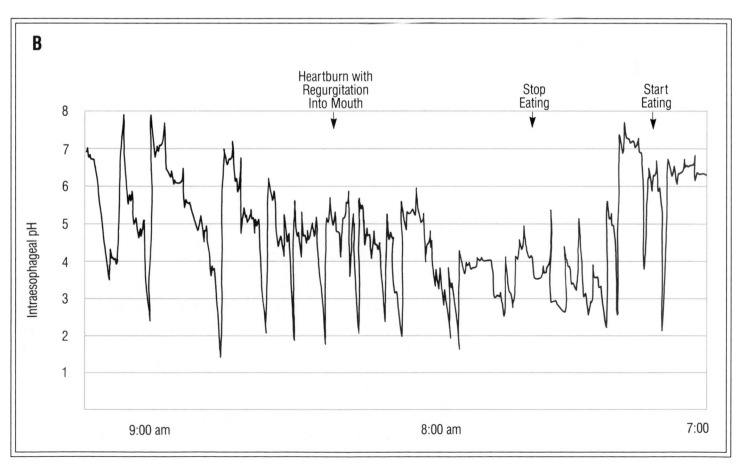

Figure 76A and B. Intraesophageal pH recording in a normal subject (A) and in a subject with GERD (B). Adapted from Demeester, et al, *Ann Surg,* 1976;184(4):463.

Therefore, since virtually everyone has acid reflux at some time during the day, other factors must affect the widespread development of acid reflux disease. Other factors include the resident time of the acid refluxed into the esophagus, levels of abdominal pressure, and the volume and toxicity of gastric contents. Under normal conditions the esophagus is able to clear acid by secondary peristalsis (Figure 77). In the presence of esophageal motor disorders, the contractions may be of low amplitude or of poor peristaltic sequencing, leading to prolonged exposure of the esophageal mucosa to acid. Salivary secretions may limit esophageal injury by buffering intraesophageal acid and by enhancing acid clearance. The secretion of saliva is impaired by radiation therapy, drugs with anticholinergic actions, and in patients with the SICCA syndrome.

A third factor in the pathogenesis of acid reflux esophagitis is the overall quantity of fluid in the stomach and the caustic nature of the gastric contents refluxed. In patients with normal gastric emptying and low acid secretion, it would be expected that only small volumes of acid would be available in the event of sphincter incompetence. In contrast, when there is delayed emptying of a large meal or acid hypersecretion for some other reason, larger quantities of free acid exist in the stomach, and this can be refluxed into the esophagus and cause damage. Furthermore, it has been suggested that in patients who have bile acid reflux into the stomach, the caustic nature of the gastric contents may be enhanced by the addition of bile.

A fifth factor involved in the pathogenesis of acid reflux disease is the decrease in local defense factors of the esophagus itself. Like the mucosa of the stomach and duodenum, the mucosa of the esophagus secretes bicarbonate from subepithelial glands and mucous. While the extent of bicarbonate secretion and mucous production is much less than that seen in the stomach and duodenum, these observations raise the possibility that mucosal defense factors are important.

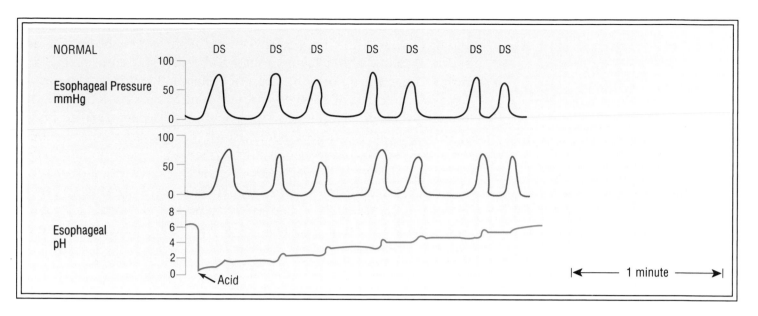

Figure 77A. Normal clearance of acid (↞) from the esophagus. (DS = Dry swallow). Pressures were measured 5 and 10 cm above the LES.

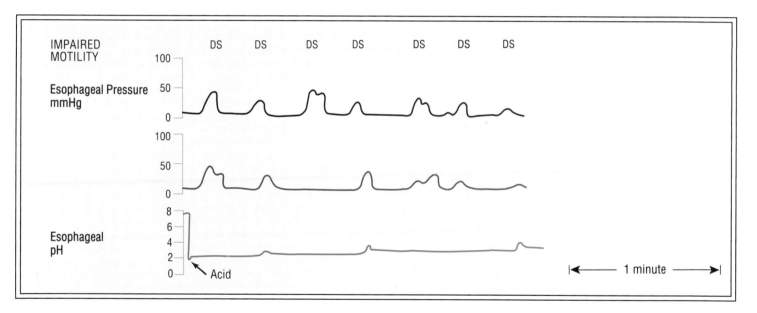

Figure 77B. Acid clearance is impaired by disordered esophageal peristalsis.

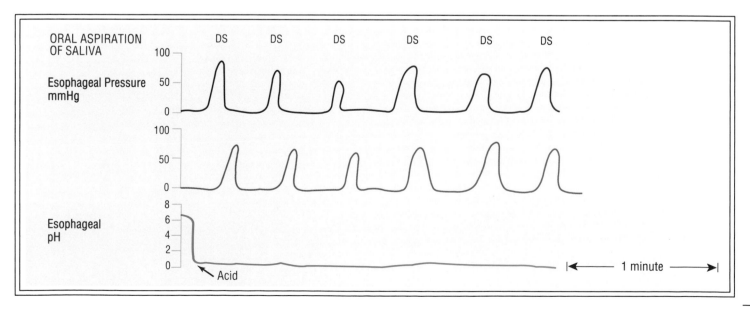

Figure 77C. Acid clearance impaired by experimental removal of saliva.

Clinical Presentation of
Gastroesophageal Reflux Disease

The most specific and frequent symptom (Figure 73) in patients with reflux disease is heartburn, defined as a burning substernal discomfort radiating from the midepigastrum. The pain may radiate into the jaw and be associated with the bitter taste of acid. The presence of a bitter taste in the back of the throat is called water brash. The symptoms of water brash, food regurgitation and heartburn become diagnostic for reflux esophagitis if they occur only in the presence of postural changes that make the esophagus dependent in relationship to the stomach. Achalasia may also present with substernal discomfort and substantial pain, described as heartburn, and with symptoms of regurgitation. In many patients it is difficult to differentiate achalasia from reflux esophagitis by history alone. Discomfort attributed to reflux must also be distinguished from infectious esophagitis, esophageal cancer, esophageal diverticuli, other forms of peptic ulcer disease, and from cardiac chest pain.

Patients with esophageal reflux often present with substernal chest discomfort, which is often thought to be cardiac in nature. Reflux may be aggravated by lifting heavy objects, which increases intra-abdominal pressure, but should not be worsened by aerobic exercise or stress. In contrast, lying down will aggravate reflux symptoms and improve exercise-related cardiac pain.

The historical evaluation of the patient should also determine whether the patient is having symptoms from complications. Deep ulcerations often induce painful swallowing, called odynophagia. The patient may also describe difficulty swallowing foods, dysphagia. Dysphagia is most commonly caused by peptic stricture, but an esophageal carcinoma must be excluded. Food caught in the distal esophagus may be described as "hanging up" in the lower chest area. Occasionally, symptoms from a distal obstruction are referred to the upper pharynx. Rarely, the patient may also experience other complications of chronic reflux esophagitis including anemia, melena, or hematemesis.

Pulmonary complications of chronic acid reflux described above may also be a presenting symptom. These pulmonary symptoms include non-allergic asthma, chronic cough and nocturnal wheezing. Many pulmonary specialists recommend complete evaluation for acid reflux disease in patients with intrinsic asthma who do not respond to bronchodilator treatment.

Radiographic and Endoscopic
Findings in Reflux Disease

Patients with symptoms of esophageal dysfunction should undergo radiographic evaluation of the upper gastrointestinal tract with particular attention towards the esophagus. When available, double contrast techniques and cinefluoroscopy should be used. The typical radiographic appearance of reflux esophagitis is shown in Figure 78.

Early radiographic findings of esophagitis include spasticity, mucosal folds, and superficial ulcerations. Esophageal damage usually extends proximally from the gastroesophageal junction and is recognized radiographically as streaks or dots of barium seen against a flat mucosa. With chronic disease the mucosa may become finely nodular or granular in appearance. Recurrent ulceration can lead to scarring and a benign peptic stricture.

The radiologist may also be able to induce reflux of barium into the esophagus by placing the patient's thorax in a dependent position. This clinical observation has relatively poor sensitivity and specificity for reflux disease. Controversy surrounds the significance of a hiatal hernia. It is clear that patients who have chronic reflux disease may develop scarring and foreshortening of the esophagus, which induces a hiatal hernia. The use of artificial maneuvers to induce a hiatal hernia during an examination may result in interesting radiographic findings but probably has little clinical significance. The lower esophageal sphincter pressures in patients with or without hiatal hernias are similar.

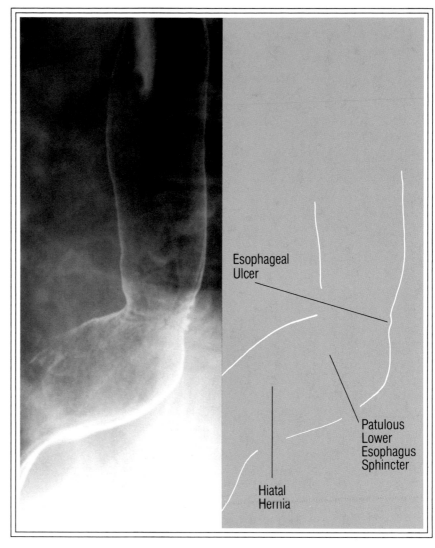

Figure 78. Radiographic appearance of peptic esophagitis. Radiograph provided by I. Laufer.

The endoscopic findings in patients with reflux esophagitis are shown in Figure 79. Here the linear ulcerations and punctate hemorrhages suggested by the X-ray are seen directly. The mucosa must be examined closely for the presence of other complications of reflux disease, including ulcerations, bleeding, friability, or Barrett's metaplasia, as discussed below. Commonly, however, the mucosa appears normal or slightly erythematous. When grossly normal, a mucosal biopsy may help to secure a diagnosis of reflux esophagitis (Figure 80). A variety of histological findings have been described in patients with acid reflux disease, but the most consistent finding is the presence of increased Rete pegs and epithelial cell hyperplasia. Epithelial hyperplasia accompanied by acute inflammation makes a diagnosis of reflux esophagitis relatively secure. Increased mucosal eosinophils may be a diagnostic histologic feature of reflux in children.

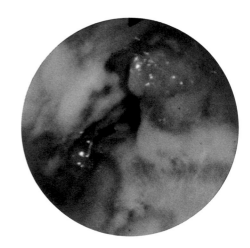

Figure 79. Endoscopic appearance of ulcerative reflux esophagitis. Endoscopy provided by J.C. Reynolds.

Patients with classic heartburn and no complications seen by upper GI examination or endoscopy need no further evaluation. When there are definitive findings of acid peptic disease on either the upper GI examination or endoscopy, further diagnostic studies are unlikely to contribute to the patient's care. More typically, however, the diagnosis remains uncertain after both evaluations, and further studies are necessary. Patients who are being considered for surgical treatment should be further examined by esophageal manometry, a Bernstein study (Figure 81), and an acid reflux test (Figure 82).

Esophageal manometry is performed by passing a pressure-sensing catheter into the esophageal lumen (Figures 81 and 82). After anesthetizing the posterior pharynx with a local anesthetic, the catheter is swallowed by the patient until all recording sites are in the stomach. The catheter is then withdrawn in a stepwise fashion to determine resting lower esophageal sphincter pressure and esophageal peristalsis at different levels. The catheter is then positioned so that the pH-sensing device is 5 cm above the lower esophageal sphincter as up to 300 mL of 0.1 N HCl is infused. If acid reflux does not occur, the study is normal. Acid clearance is determined from the number of swallows necessary to increase the pH to normal (Figures 77 and 82). Therefore, through this single examination, basal lower esophageal pressure, the orderliness of peristalsis in the esophageal body, and the effectiveness of the barrier to prevent acid reflux are determined. Furthermore, one can determine whether the presence of refluxed acid mimics the patient's primary complaint and, finally, whether the patient is able to clear acid from the esophagus. Following this single examination the physiological abnormalities causing reflux are usually apparent.

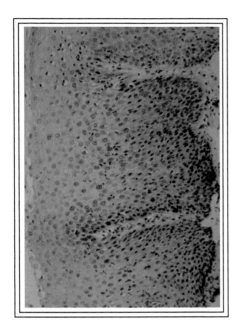

Figure 80. Histology of GERD. Photograph provided by S.H. Saul.

Figure 81. Technique for esophageal manometry and the Bernstein test.

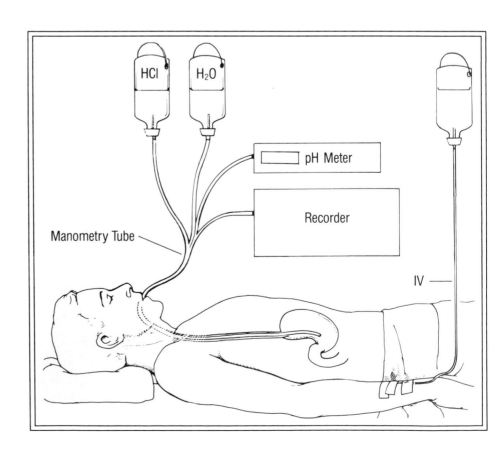

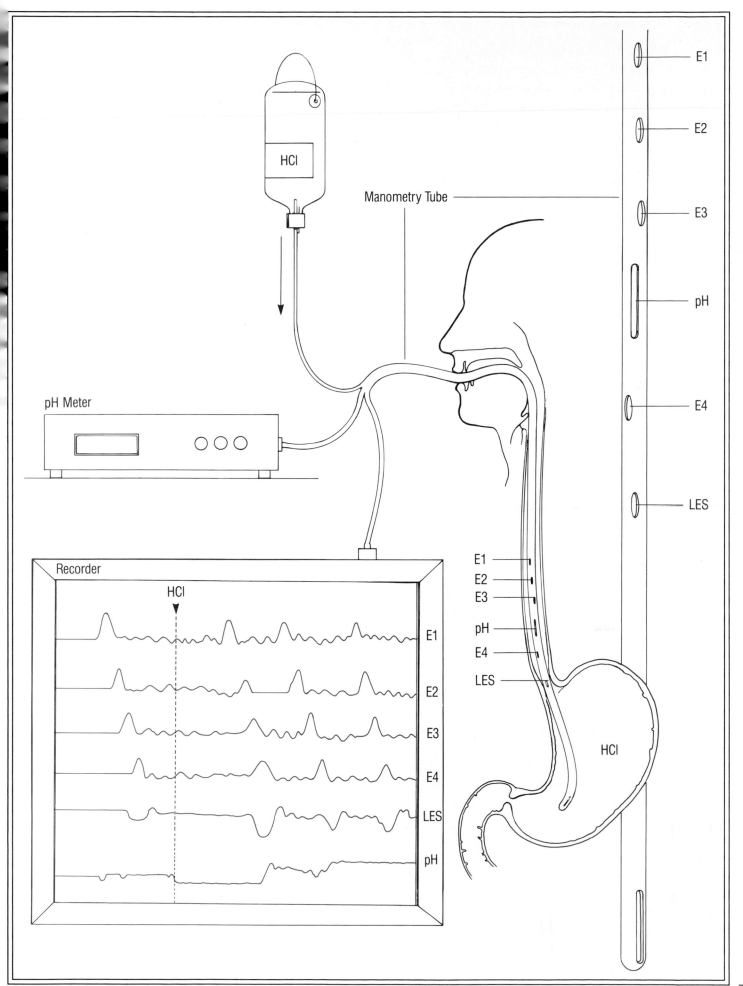

Figure 82. Standard acid reflux test. A bolus infusion of HCl into the stomach is associated with a fall in intraesophageal pH. Pressures at and above the lower esophageal sphincter (LES) are also determined.

Rarely, even after all of these studies further evaluation is necessary. For this reason 24-hour pH recordings have been developed (Figure 76). Computer-assisted analyses allow one to determine the time during which the esophagus is exposed to acid. The number of reflux episodes and the correlation between reflux episodes and the patient's symptoms can also be determined over a 24-hour period (Figure 83). Such studies are extremely valuable in the analysis of drug therapy and surgery but are not necessary in the vast majority of patients with heartburn. Questions have been raised about the specificity of the study and the need for a full 24-hour recording. Several authors have suggested that the recording time may be decreased to 8 hours if it includes many of the patient's normal activities, including lying down, sleeping, and eating several meals. Further determination of the importance and need for such prolonged recordings in the evaluation and treatment of patients with reflux disease is underway.

Complications of Gastroesophageal Reflux Disease

Esophageal Complications: The most common complication of acid reflux disease is intractable pain. The correlation between pain and esophageal mucosal findings during radiographic or endoscopic evaluation is poor. Many patients complain of intractable symptoms when morphologic studies show minimal abnormalities. It is in such patients that further evaluations with standard reflux acid test, manometry, and perhaps prolonged intraesophageal pH recordings are necessary. When the duration of acid reflux or the frequency of reflux episodes is not significantly greater than normal or when the reflux barrier is shown to be intact by the standard acid reflux test, the diagnosis of a supersensitive esophagus may be more appropriate than proceeding with surgical intervention. In these patients, psychotherapy and psychopharmaceuticals may be a valuable adjunct to the usual therapeutic interventions.

Figure 83. Quantitative acid reflux in normal subjects and in patients with esophagitis and Barrett's metaplasia.

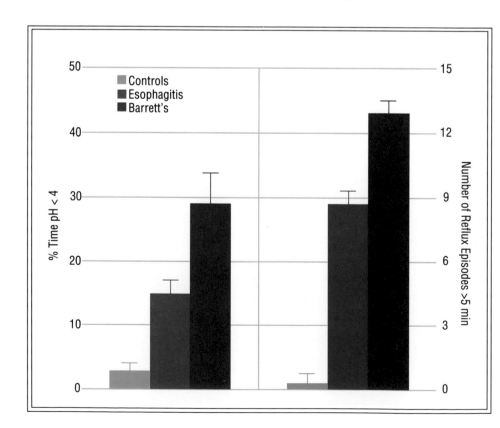

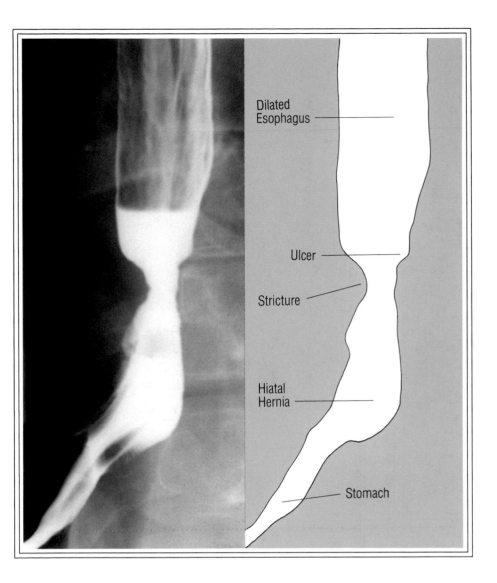

Figure 84. Esophageal stricture. Radiograph provided by I. Lauber.

Obstruction occurs in patients with chronic reflux esophagitis when recurrent ulcerations scar down to form strictures (Figure 84). These strictures typically occur in the distal third of the esophagus. Strictures lead to difficulty swallowing foods, with solids being more difficult than liquids. Symptoms are usually referred to the position of obstruction, but, not uncommonly, symptoms are referred instead to the cervical esophagus. The vast majority of such strictures can be handled medically and dilated pneumatically or with bougienage.

Bleeding frequently occurs in patients with severe gastroesophageal reflux disease, although the volumes of blood lost are usually small. Rarely, a patient will present with hematemesis, but more typically there will be guaiac-positive stools of normal color. Iron deficiency anemia is not uncommon. Endoscopically one finds deep ulcerations, active bleeding, or mucosal friability in these subjects (Figure 85).

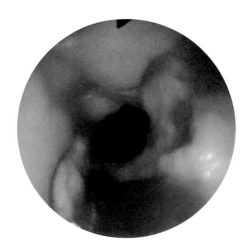

Figure 85. Bleeding esophageal ulcerations. Endoscopy provided by J.C. Reynolds.

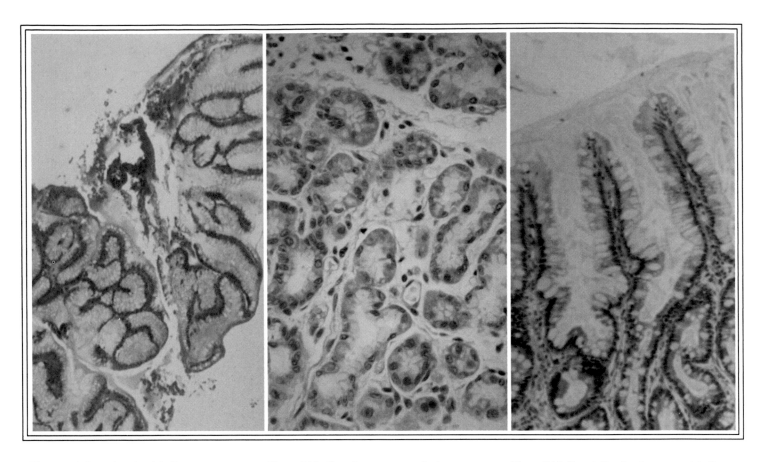

Figure 86A. Junctional epithelium.　　　　*Figure 86B*. Gastric type metaplasia.　　　　*Figure 86C*. Specialized columnar epithelium.

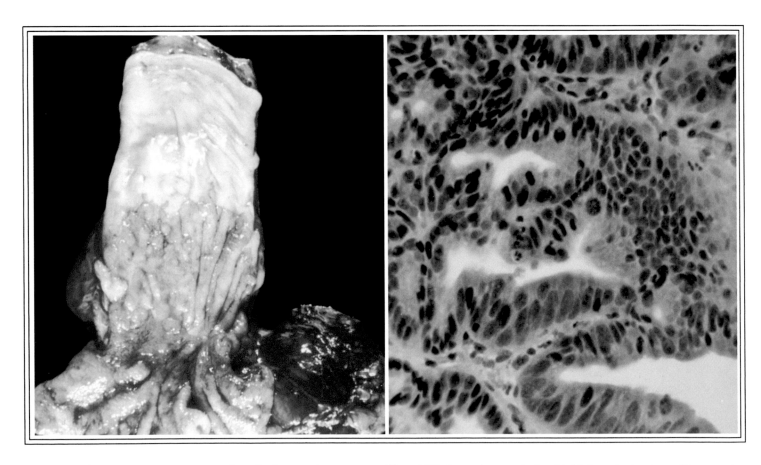

Figure 86D. Gross anatomic appearance of small adenocarcinoma arising in Barrett's esophagus.

Figure 86E. Barrett's metaplasia with high grade dysplasia. Photographs for Figures 86 A-E provided by S.H. Saul.

The most serious complication of chronic acid reflux disease is Barrett's metaplasia, a replacement of the normal squamous epithelium of the esophagus by columnar epithelium. This metaplastic transformation occurs as one of three histologic patterns (Figure 86 A-C). It has been estimated that 3% to 7% of patients with such metaplastic change will undergo carcinomatous transformation at some time in their life (Figure 86 D,E). Such patients require close scrutiny and surveillance by biopsies to detect change from metaplasia to dysplasia. These patients invariably have severe acid reflux, very low LES pressures, and prolonged exposure to acid on 24-hour ambulatory pH studies (Figure 83). Maximal therapy is clearly indicated in these patients.

Pulmonary Complications: As discussed above, pulmonary complications are being noted with increased frequency in patients with gastroesophageal reflux disease. These include aspiration pneumonia, interstitial lung disease, asthma, nocturnal cough, or wheezing. The importance of gastroesophageal reflux as a cause of nosocomial pneumonia, particularly in patients with intrinsic or therapeutically induced achlorhydria, is also being recognized as a very serious and all-too-common complication of nasogastric intubation in patients with impaired gag reflex.

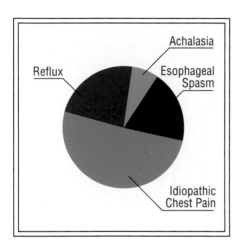

Figure 87. Relative incidence of causes of noncardiac chest pain.

Chest Pain: Gastroesophageal reflux is an important cause of noncardiac chest pain (Figure 87). Patients with reflux, with or without spasm, are responsible for up to 50% of all catheter-negative anginal pain syndromes. The diagnosis of an esophageal cause for chest pain can significantly improve the quality of life of a patient who fears that his recurrent pain is cardiac in nature.

RECOMMENDED READING

1. Soll AH, Isenberg J: Duodenal ulcer diseases, in Sleisenger MH, Fordtran JS (eds): *Gastrointestinal Disease: Pathophysiology Diagnosis Management,* ed 3. Philadelphia, WB Saunders Co, 1983, vol 1, chap 40.

2. Richardson CT: Gastric ulcer, in Sleisinger MH, Fordtran JS (eds): *Gastrointestinal Disease: Pathophysiology Diagnosis Management,* ed 3. Philadelphia, WB Saunders Co, 1983, vol 1, chap 41.

3. Robert A, Kauffman GL Jr: Stress ulcers, in Sleisinger MH, Fordtran JS (eds): *Gastrointestinal Disease: Pathophysiology Diagnosis Management,* ed 3. Philadelphia, WB, Saunders Co, 1983, vol 1, chap 39.

4. Dodds WJ, Hogan WJ, Helm JF, Dent J: Pathogenesis of reflux esophagitis. *Gastroenterology* 1981;81:376-394.

5. Dodds WJ, Dent J, Hogan WJ, et al: Mechanisms of gastroesophageal reflux in patients with reflux esophagitis. *N Engl J Med* 1962;307:1547-1552.

6. Katz PO, Dalton CD, Richter JE, et al: Esophageal testing of patients with non cardiac chest pain or dysphagia. Results of three years' experience with 1161 patients. *Ann Intern Med* 1987;106:593-597.

Arthur J. Atkinson, Jr., M.D.
and Robert M. Craig, M.D.

Principles of Management

GOALS FOR TREATING PATIENTS
WITH ACID-PEPTIC DISEASE

Relieve Pain

Promote Healing

Prevent Recurrence

Prevent Complications

Hemorrhage

Obstruction

Perforation

Figure 88. Goals for treating patients with acid-peptic disease.

The immediate goals of therapy for patients who present with symptoms of uncomplicated acid-peptic disease are to provide effective pain relief, to promote healing, and to prevent recurrence and the development of the complications of hemorrhage, obstruction, and perforation (Figure 88). A common characteristic of reflux esophagitis, gastric ulcer, and duodenal ulcer is the tendency for these conditions to recur. Accordingly, initial therapy needs to be followed by a long-term management program designed to decrease the recurrence of symptomatic disease and of asymptomatic recurrences, which for ulcers may be more frequent than symptomatic recurrences. Even though much remains to be learned about underlying pathophysiologic mechanisms, it is clear that acid-peptic disease, in general terms, represents an imbalance between aggressive and defensive factors in the upper gastrointestinal tract. The goal of therapeutic interventions is to reset this balance either by reducing mucosal exposure to acid or by bolstering cytoprotection.

Before turning to specific pharmacotherapy, it is appropriate to consider several general measures that should be instituted promptly and maintained indefinitely in managing patients with acid-peptic disease. Patients with reflux esophagitis should avoid anything that promotes acid reflux by relaxing the lower esophageal sphincter. This includes smoking, use of alcohol, and ingestion of large meals, which cause gastric distention. Since a horizontal position also facilitates reflux of gastric contents into the esophagus, patients should not lie down immediately after eating. They may also benefit from sleeping on a bed that is tilted by placing blocks under the head. Consumption of coffee, with or without caffeine, should be moderate, and greasy or spicy foods should be avoided.

In patients with peptic ulcer disease, cigarette smoking should be prohibited since it retards ulcer healing and increases the risk of relapse of duodenal and gastric ulcers. The precise mechanism by which smoking impairs ulcer healing has not been established. Cigarette smoking increases basal acid secretion, decreases inhibition of nocturnal acid secretion by H_2-receptor antagonists, and appears to increase the risk of recurrence (Figure 89). Accordingly, cessation of smoking may be even more important than drug therapy in treating patients with ulcer disease. Alcohol should be allowed only in moderation. Administration of milk and restriction of diet are time-honored measures that appear to provide some patients with symptomatic relief but have not been shown to accelerate ulcer healing. On the other hand, aspirin and other nonsteroidal anti-inflammatory drugs (NSAIDs) may precipitate or exacerbate a gastric ulcer. There is inconclusive evidence that these agents can adversely affect duodenal ulcers, but since they are generally injurious to the mucosa of the upper gastrointestinal tract, their use should be minimized. High doses of adrenal cortical steroids increase the incidence of both gastric and duodenal ulcers and should be avoided if possible.

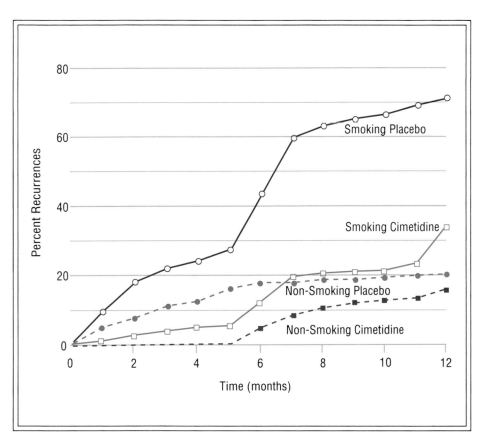

Figure 89. Recurrence of symptomatic and endoscopically verified asymptomatic duodenal ulcers. Adapted from Sontag, et al, *N Engl J Med,* 1984;311:689-693.

Pharmacotherapeutic Modalities

Antacid Therapy

Rationale

A variety of pharmacologic agents are useful in treating patients with acid-peptic disease (Figure 90). These include antacids, inhibitors of acid secretion, cytoprotective agents, and prokinetic agents.

The function of antacids is to neutralize the hydrochloric acid secreted by gastric parietal cells. Commonly used antacids differ in terms of their composition and *acid neutralizing capacity* (ANC) (Figure 91). ANC is defined as the number of milliequivalents of 1 N HCl that can be brought *in vitro* to pH 3.5 in 15 minutes. The time limit is imposed because, in the absence of food, some antacid compounds, most notably aluminum hydroxide, neutralize gastric acid at a rate slower than that of gastric emptying. Clinical efficacy generally parallels ANC, but some deviation occurs because nucleoproteins and other gastric contents may selectively slow acid neutralization by some compounds.

Antacids have been the traditional approach for treatment of patients with reflux esophagitis, and clinical experience suggests that they provide

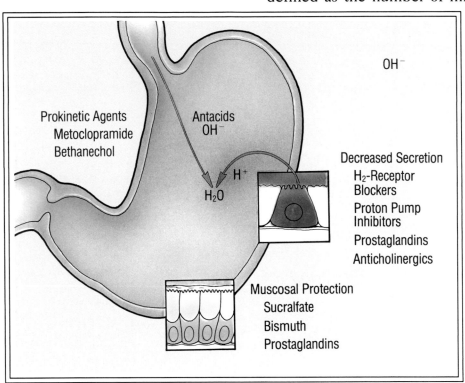

Figure 90. Pharmacologic agents used to treat acid-peptic disease.

Figure 91. Properties of some commonly used antacid formulations.

PRODUCT	ACID NEUTRALIZING CAPACITY (mEq/5 ml or tablet)	CaCO₃	Al(OH)₃	Mg(OH)₂	Na	SIMETHICONE
LIQUID SUSPENSIONS						
Alternagel	16	0	600	0	2.5	0
Amphojel	10	0	320	0	0.1	0
Delcid	42	0	600	665	15.0	0
Gelusil-II	24	0	400	400	1.3	30
Maalox	13	0	225	200	1.3	0
Maalox-TC	27	0	600	300	0.8	0
Milk of Magnesia	14	0	0	388	0.12	0
Mylanta	13	0	200	200	0.7	20
Mylanta-II	25	0	600	300	1.1	20
Riopan	15	0	*	*	<0.1	0
Titralac Plus	11	500	0	0	0	20
TABLETS						
Maalox-TC	28	0	600	300	0.5	0
Rolaids	7.5	0	325 mg NaAl(CO₃)(OH)₂	0	53.0	0
Tums	10	500	0	0	2.0	0

The CONTENT columns are measured in mg/5 ml or tablet.

*Riopan contains 540 mg magaldrate, a complex hydroxymagnesium aluminate.

relief of gastric and duodenal ulcer pain. There is evidence that antacid therapy also accelerates the healing of gastric and duodenal ulcers. In addition, antacids used in relatively large quantities have been found to be effective in preventing stress-induced bleeding in critically ill patients.

Antacids share a number of secondary effects that influence their therapeutic utility. Partial neutralization of gastric acid may paradoxically increase peptic activity since gastric pepsin has maximal activity at a pH of 2 to 3, and substantial activity is seen until gastric pH is raised above 4 (Figure 47). This may necessitate administering seven daily doses of a strong antacid with a total ANC of at least 50 to 80 milliequivalents (Figure 92). The timing of administration of antacids is particularly important since antacids taken on an empty stomach quickly pass through to the duodenum, and their effects are of short duration. Thus, the acid neutralizing ability of antacids is optimized when doses are administered 1 and 3 hours postprandially and before bed.

Although most products have relatively similar ANC, their chemical composition differs widely and affects their therapeutic utility (Figure 91). Sodium bicarbonate, in the form of baking soda, is commonly employed as a home remedy for indigestion. The chemical reactions that sodium bicarbonate and other antacids undergo in the stomach are summarized in Figure 93. Not only is sodium bicarbonate rapidly emptied from the stomach because of its water solubility, but it is unsuitable for repeated use because it is readily absorbed and can cause metabolic alkalosis. Its high sodium content may also promote fluid retention.

Chemical Composition of Antacid Products

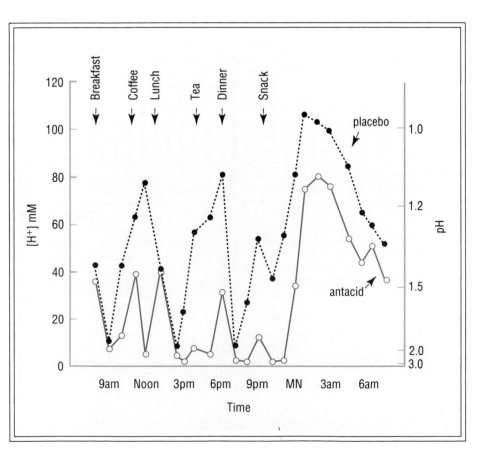

Figure 92. Reduction of intragastric pH by antacids. Adapted from Milton-Thompson, in *Antacids in the Eighties,* 1982. Antacid is administered 1 and 3 hours postprandially and before bed.

Calcium carbonate is perhaps the most potent acid neutralizing compound. However, calcium-containing antacids may cause a paradoxical rebound in gastric acid secretion. Further, absorption of calcium chloride (Figure 93) may be sufficient to precipitate the milk-alkali syndrome. In addition, release of carbon dioxide causes abdominal distention and belching that may exacerbate reflux esophagitis.

Aluminum hydroxide is relatively insoluble in water and polymerizes to a number of products that neutralize gastric acid at different rates. This compound has relatively limited efficacy and, even when most reactive, neutralizes acid too slowly to elevate gastric pH much above 4.5. Aluminum hydroxide delays gastric emptying, and this may promote its activity as an antacid. However, aluminum-containing compounds retard intestinal motility and may be excessively constipating, particularly in elderly patients. Aluminum chloride, the product of the reaction of aluminum hydroxide and hydrochloric acid (Figure 93) is poorly absorbed, but plasma concentrations of aluminum are likely to be elevated in patients with renal failure who receive long-term therapy with aluminum-containing antacids.

Magnesium hydroxide is the most rapidly acting of the insoluble antacids, and magnesium chloride, the reaction product, is poorly absorbed (Figure 93). The insolubility of magnesium hydroxide may slow its removal from the stomach and prolong its duration of action. However, a general characteristic of magnesium-containing compounds is that they increase intestinal motility.

Accordingly, the primary rationale for including mixtures of aluminum and magnesium hydroxide in commercial formulations is to offset the adverse effects on intestinal motility that would be observed if either compound were given by itself. Magaldrate is a hydroxymagnesium aluminate complex that is rapidly converted by hydrochloric acid to magnesium ion and aluminum hydroxide. Administration of magaldrate results in a balanced effect on intestinal motility, and there is not sufficient time for the aluminum hydroxide that is generated in the presence of gastric acid to be converted to less active derivatives. This results in a more effective antacid action than would be obtained with simple physical mixtures of the hydroxides.

Many commercial antacid formulations also contain simethicone (Figure 91), a surface-active agent that may decrease foam. The sodium content of antacids is also a concern for patients with

Figure 93. Chemical reactions of antacid compounds with gastric acid.*

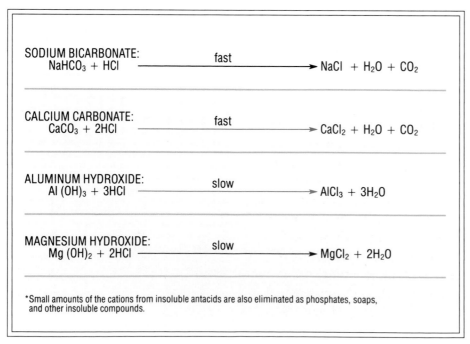

SODIUM BICARBONATE:
$NaHCO_3 + HCl$ —— fast ——→ $NaCl + H_2O + CO_2$

CALCIUM CARBONATE:
$CaCO_3 + 2HCl$ —— fast ——→ $CaCl_2 + H_2O + CO_2$

ALUMINUM HYDROXIDE:
$Al(OH)_3 + 3HCl$ —— slow ——→ $AlCl_3 + 3H_2O$

MAGNESIUM HYDROXIDE:
$Mg(OH)_2 + 2HCl$ —— slow ——→ $MgCl_2 + 2H_2O$

*Small amounts of the cations from insoluble antacids are also eliminated as phosphates, soaps, and other insoluble compounds.

hypertension or individuals who suffer from fluid retention due to cardiac or renal disease. A number of antacid products have now been developed that contain less than 1.0 mg of sodium per 5 ml.

The effect of therapy with antacids on bowel motility is a major concern and is largely responsible for the inclusion of both aluminum and magnesium in many proprietary mixtures. In fact, milk of magnesia is widely used by the lay public and in hospital practice as a laxative. The constipating effects of aluminum hydroxide are proportional to the administered dose and have rarely resulted in ileus and bowel perforation. Calcium carbonate usually has constipating effects but occasionally may cause diarrhea.

Antacids exert a stimulating effect on gastric acid secretion, and *acid rebound*, defined as sustained hypersecretion of gastric acid after the ingestion of an antacid, may limit the efficacy of therapy with an antacid in some patients. Although sodium bicarbonate and the hydroxides of aluminum and magnesium can all stimulate secretion of gastric acid, calcium carbonate is particularly likely to cause an exaggerated and sustained rebound in gastric acid secretion. This apparently specific action of calcium is partly mediated by release of gastrin and partly reflects direct stimulation of parietal cells. Thus, calcium compounds are infrequently used as antacids, even though calcium carbonate has the highest potency in neutralizing gastric acid.

The *milk-alkali syndrome* is another complication of antacid therapy that was seen when frequent, large doses of sodium bicarbonate and/or calcium carbonate were administered with milk or cream to patients with peptic ulcer disease. Therapeutic regimens emphasizing the use of dairy products are seldom employed in current practice. This syndrome, precipitated by systemic absorption of sodium bicarbonate and calcium chloride (Figure 93), was especially threatening to patients with impaired renal function. In milk-alkali syndrome, symptoms of hypercalcemia, including weakness, lethargy, mental confusion, anorexia, nausea, and vomiting, which exacerbates a metabolic alkalosis, occur, usually within 3-8 days of initiating therapy. Convulsions and death are occasional sequelae.

Finally, a secondary effect that influences the therapeutic utility of antacids results from the fact that even though those containing magnesium and aluminum are relatively safe, the alkalosis that results from their chronic use predisposes patients to nephrolithiasis. In addition, absorption of aluminum-containing antacids may cause osteoporosis, proximal myopathy and encephalopathy in patients with impaired renal function. Antacids also have been shown to reduce the bioavailability of a number of drugs, including digoxin, cimetidine, and ranitidine, and to form non-absorbable chelates with iron and tetracycline. However, patient acceptance remains the major limitation of antacid therapy since the rapidity of gastric emptying necessitates an intensive regimen in which doses of antacid are administered seven times daily (Figure 92). This inconvenience is partly ameliorated by the availability of solid dosage forms for many preparations of antacids (Figure 91).

Limitations and Complications

88

Drugs Blocking Acid Secretion

Blockade of acid secretion is currently the most useful therapeutic strategy in treating patients with acid-peptic disease. *In vitro* studies have demonstrated that parietal cells have specific receptors for each of several stimuli of gastric acid secretion, including histamine, acetylcholine, and gastrin (Figure 94). Histamine acts through H_2-receptors and the stimulation of adenylate cyclase activity to stimulate secretory activity. It also acts indirectly to amplify the stimulatory effects of acetylcholine and gastrin. Therapy with H_2-receptor antagonists not only provides a competitive, dose-dependent antagonism of the effects of histamine stimulation but also blunts responses to cholinergic stimuli and gastrin. Anticholinergic drugs bind to muscarinic receptors on parietal cells and can inhibit basal and nocturnal acid secretion by 40%-50%, vagal stimulated secretion by 50%-70%, and postprandial secretion by 30%-40%. Gastrin is a relatively weak stimulant of gastric acid secretion. The gastrin-receptor antagonist, proglumide, has only limited efficacy in reducing secretion of gastric acid. Prostaglandin E_2 and its analogs bind to receptors on parietal cells and suppress gastric acid secretion by activating a guanine nucleotide-binding regulatory protein (G_i) that inhibits histamine-stimulated adenylate cyclase activity. Naturally occurring prostaglandins are quickly degraded in the gastrointestinal tract and are only effective when given parenterally. On the other hand, methylated analogs can be given orally and have clinical utility. The final common pathway in gastric acid secretion is activation of an H^+-K^+-adenosinetriphosphatase (ATPase) that is located on the secretory canalicular surface of parietal cells. This enzyme is unique to the gastric mucosa and functions as a proton pump. Blockade of this pump by benzimidazole derivatives results in a profound and sustained suppression of gastric acid secretion.

The introduction of H_2-receptor blocking drugs has dramatically altered the treatment of acid-peptic disease and has opened new vistas in understanding the pharmacology of histamine. For example, a 300 mg dose of cimetidine typically reduces basal acid secretion by more than 90% for 4 hours and inhibits meal-stimulated acid secretion by about 70% for 3 hours. The clinical utility of H_2-receptor antagonists has been so well established that these agents have become among the most widely used drugs in the world.

Although the structure of the H_2-receptor has not been determined and rigorous structure-activity relationships have not been established for H_2-receptor blocking drugs, most effective compounds include a heterocyclic aromatic ring with a flexible side-chain that is joined to a non-ionizable polar group that has marked hydrogen-binding properties (Figure 95). H_2-receptor blocking drugs act as competitive antagonists of histamine, and their effects are reversible and relatively short-lived. The imidazole ring of histamine apparently binds to the H_2-receptor at a specific site, and this is the presumed point of attachment of the aromatic ring of H_2-blocking drugs. The rest of the molecule contributes additional binding energy by interacting with accessory regions of the receptor, as indicated by the fact that side-chain length is an important determinant of the potency of H_2 antagonists. In contrast to anti-adrenergic, anticholinergic, and H_1-receptor blockers that incorporate lipophilic substituents to enhance their binding to receptor sites, H_2-receptor blockers are hydrophilic molecules, and it is likely that their interaction with H_2-receptors is primarily mediated by hydrogen bonding.

H_2-Receptor Blocking Drugs

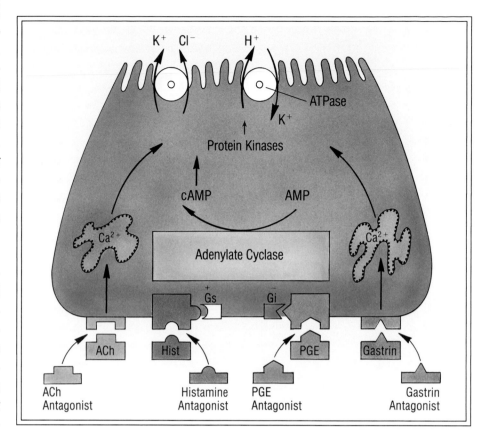

Figure 94. Schematic representation of parietal cell showing pathways through which secretagogues stimulate secretion of hydrogen ions.

Basis for Therapeutic Activity

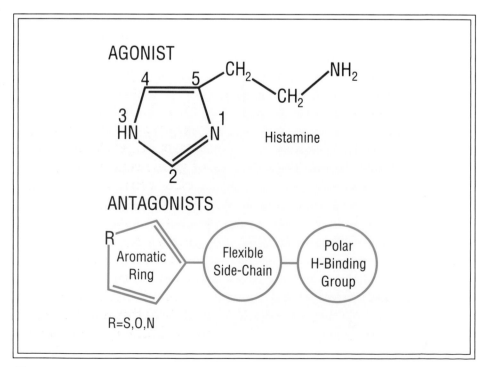

Figure 95. Structure of histamine and the prototypic structure of an H_2 antagonist showing multiple domains.

Compounds with antihistaminic activity were first discovered by Bovet and colleagues in 1937, but these compounds, now known as H_1-receptor antagonists, did not inhibit histamine-stimulated gastric acid secretion. In 1964, Black began a systematic program in which histamine was used as a starting point to design molecules that would bind more tightly than histamine at histamine receptors without triggering the usual acid secretory response. Over 200 compounds were synthesized and tested before N^α-guanylhistamine was identified as a compound that bound to H_2-receptors but had only weak activity as an agonist at these receptors (Figure 96). The affinity of H_2-receptors for these agents was enhanced by lengthening the side-chain, but stimulatory activity was lost only when the strongly basic amidine side-chain was replaced by a polar, but uncharged, basic functional group. Burimamide, synthesized with a thiourea side-chain, was the first compound shown to be a specific antagonist of histamine at H_2-receptors, but clinical trials indicated that it lacked sufficient potency to have therapeutic utility. Potency was increased by adding a methyl group at the 4-position of the imidazole ring and by substituting sulfur for one of the side-chain carbon atoms to form metiamide (Figure 96). However, clinical trials of metiamide were discontinued when it was found to cause granulocytopenia in some patients. This side effect was attributed to the thiourea side-chain group. Replacement of the thiourea sulfur atom with a cyanoimmino group resulted in cimetidine, the first clinically useful H_2-receptor antagonist.

Although the first H_2-receptor blocking drugs all incorporated the imidazole ring of histamine, this is not a prerequisite for activity. Newer drugs incorporate a variety of aromatic rings (Figure 97), and it has been suggested that these compounds be classified according to the chemical structure of this ring. Most of these newer agents have greater potency as H_2-receptor antagonists than cimetidine although it has not been shown that greater potency yields any additional clinical benefit. Recommended doses of the various H_2 antagonists result in acid suppression to a similar extent and have similar clinical efficacy.

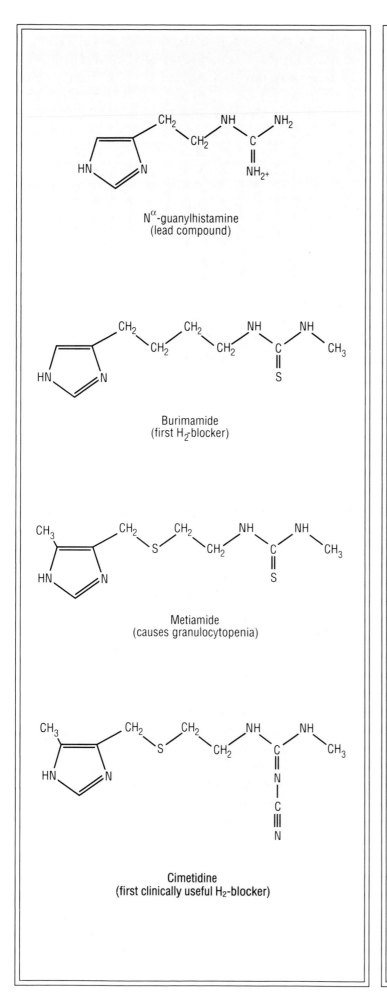

Figure 96. Development of H₂ antagonists.

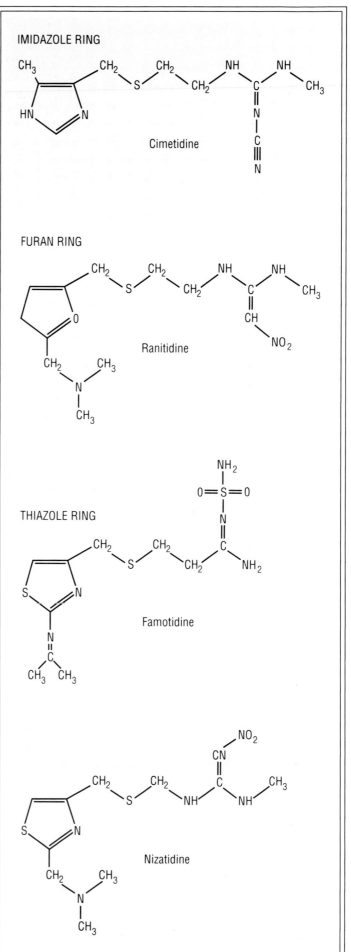

Figure 97. Aromatic rings used in H₂ antagonists.

Extensive clinical experience with cimetidine and ranitidine and more limited experience with famotidine and nizatidine have established that adverse reactions to these drugs are infrequent and, generally, of minor clinical significance. In contrast to effects observed following administration of other classes of receptor antagonists, the adverse reactions that occur in patients taking H_2 antagonists are rarely due to an action at the receptor. Constipation, diarrhea, skin rash, and dizziness are idiosyncratic side effects that have been reported as rare complications of therapy with these drugs. The incidence of these side effects is frequently similar to that observed following administration of a placebo. Transient elevations in serum aminotransferase levels and hepatic injury have been reported to occur in isolated cases. Small increases in serum creatinine concentration may occur after initiating therapy with cimetidine or ranitidine. This does not usually indicate nephrotoxicity and presumably reflects competition between cimetidine or ranitidine and creatinine for renal tubular secretion. Severe headaches have been reported in 3%-6% of patients taking ranitidine. Headaches have also been reported in patients being treated with famotidine. This effect does not appear to be associated with inhibition of H_2-receptors. Dose-related side effects of therapy with H_2-receptor antagonists, including lethargy, agitation, mental confusion, and coma, have been observed. These side effects have usually been reported in patients who are elderly or who have impaired hepatic function or ulcers associated with hypergastrinemic states which, like Zollinger-Ellison syndrome, require unusually high doses of an H_2-receptor antagonist. Cimetidine elevates serum prolactin levels and binds to androgen receptors. Gynecomastia and decreased sexual drive have been reported. These effects occur when daily doses of cimetidine in excess of 3 gm are used as may be required in patients with Zollinger-Ellison syndrome.

Extensive studies of the drug-drug interactions seen with H_2 antagonists have led to an increased understanding of the mechanisms of hepatic and renal clearance of a variety of agents. Cimetidine may interfere with nonrenal drug elimination by Type II binding to cytochrome P-450. Ranitidine binds less tightly to cytochrome P-450 and would not be expected to be as likely as cimetidine to interfere with the function of hepatic microsomal enzymes, although interactions with warfarin and theophylline have been reported. Nizatidine binds weakly and current, though limited data suggest that famotidine does not bind at all to the cytochrome P-450 system, and these drugs are less likely to cause significant interactions with drugs undergoing hepatic metabolism.

Inhibition of renal tubular secretion of drugs such as procainamide has been seen with both cimetidine and ranitidine. Because of its greater therapeutic potency, ranitidine is given in lower doses and may be less likely than cimetidine to interfere with renal tubular drug excretion.

Product-	IC$_{50}$* ng/ml	Oral Absorption %	V$_{d(area)}$ L/kg	Cl$_E$ ml/min	T$_{1/2}$ hr	Renal Excretion %
Cimetidine	780	62	1.8	583	1.9	77
Ranitidine	165	50-60	1.8	709	2.1	69
Famotidine	13	37	1.3	400	2.6	72
Nizatidine	84	95	1.2	767	1.3	78

*Plasma concentration needed to inhibit gastric acid secretion by 50%.

Figure 98. Pharmacokinetic properties of H$_2$-receptor antagonists in normal subjects.

The relationship between plasma concentration and inhibition of gastric acid secretion has been elucidated for H$_2$-receptor antagonists, and the approximate concentrations required to inhibit acid secretion by 50% (IC$_{50}$) have been determined (Figure 98). However, there is little information about the degree of inhibition of gastric acid secretion required to promote healing in patients with peptic ulcer disease, and routine plasma level monitoring has not been found to be useful.

The H$_2$-receptor antagonists presently available have similar pharmacokinetic properties (Figure 98). With the exception of nizatidine, less than half to two thirds of an oral dose is usually absorbed. In the case of cimetidine, bioavailability has been shown to be formulation-dependent. Bioavailability has generally been evaluated in normal volunteers, and it is possible that absorption of these compounds may be sufficiently compromised in certain types of patients to account for therapeutic failure. For example, delayed or decreased absorption of cimetidine and ranitidine may account for the high oral dose requirements of some patients with Zollinger-Ellison syndrome. Binding to plasma proteins ranges from 15% to 30%, and these compounds are distributed in an apparent volume that exceeds total body water. Renal tubular secretion of these drugs can be inferred from the fact that their renal clearance (Cl$_E$ x % renal excretion) exceeds the glomerular filtration rate. Since these agents are excreted primarily by the kidneys, dosage should be reduced when treating patients with impaired renal function.

Pharmacokinetics of H$_2$-Receptor Antagonists

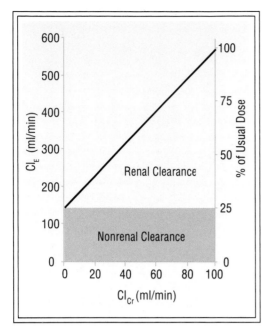

Figure 99. Relationship between creatinine clearance (Cl_{Cr}), cimetidine elimination clearance (Cl_E), and appropriate cimetidine dose reduction for patients with impaired renal function.

Recognition of impaired renal function can be a particular problem in elderly patients in whom a decreased skeletal muscle mass may result in normal serum creatinine values even when renal function is markedly impaired, and the Cockroft and Gault equation can be used to estimate creatinine clearance so that appropriate dose reductions can be made.

In men, this equation provides the following estimate of creatinine clearance:

$$Cl_{Cr} = \frac{(140 - age) \cdot (weight\ in\ kg)}{72 \cdot (serum\ Cr\ in\ mg/dl)}$$

For women, this estimate should be reduced by 15%.

Since the nonrenal clearance of cimetidine is unimpaired, even in functionally anephric patients, the data in Figure 98 can be used to construct a simple nomogram to guide cimetidine dosing (Figure 99). From the nomogram, it can be estimated that a functionally anephric patient should receive one quarter of the usual cimetidine dose and that a patient with a creatinine clearance of 40 ml/min should receive half the usual dose. Similar considerations should be applied to dosing with other H_2-receptor antagonists.

Proton Pump Inhibitors

A number of benzimidazole derivatives inhibit the H^+-K^+-ATPase that functions as a proton pump and is the final common step in acid secretion by parietal cells (Figure 94). Omeprazole is the prototypic drug in this class (Figure 100). It is a weak base that diffuses from the bloodstream to the cytosol of the parietal cell and then distributes preferentially to the acidic milieu of the canalicular system where it is concentrated in the protonated form and undergoes acid catalyzed conversion to sulfenic acid and sulfenamide (Figure 101A). These compounds are permanent cations that inactivate the H^+-K^+-ATPase by forming bonds with sulfhydryl groups in the luminal sector of this enzyme. Because this inactivation is irreversible, a single dose of omeprazole results in inhibition of basal and stimulated secretion of gastric acid by more than 90% for 24 hours, even though the elimination half-life of omeprazole is less than 1 hour. Return of gastric acid secretion to pretreatment levels requires the synthesis of new molecules of H^+-K^+-ATPase.

OMEPRAZOLE
(proton pump inhibitor)

PIRENZEPINE
(antagonist of muscarinic cholinergic receptors {M_1})

MISOPROSTOL
(analog of PGE_2)

Figure 100. Drugs blocking acid secretion.

Omeprazole thus has greater efficacy than H_2-receptor blocking drugs, and administration of a single morning dose completely eliminates intragastric acidity during the late afternoon and evening when relatively poor control is provided by H_2-antagonists (Figure 101B). Omeprazole has been shown to be effective in treating patients with peptic ulcer disease and reflux esophagitis and has proved especially useful in managing patients with Zollinger-Ellison syndrome who have not responded satisfactorily to treatment with H_2-receptor antagonists. Omeprazole owes its selectivity of action to the fact that the H^+-K^+-ATPase appears to be located only in gastric parietal cells.

Relatively few side effects have been reported in trials with omeprazole. However, clinical experience with this agent is limited. It is possible that sustained gastric anacidity such as that which occurs following administration of a proton pump inhibitor may predispose to bacterial contamination of the stomach. This is a potential concern if omeprazole is used for long-term therapy since metabolism of nitrites to N-nitroso compounds by gastric bacteria has been proposed as an etiologic factor in the association of achlorhydria with gastric cancer. Carcinoid tumors have been reported in studies with omeprazole in rats. In addition, omeprazole and its sulfone metabolite bind tightly to cytochrome P-450 and have been shown to interfere with hepatic metabolism of phenytoin and diazepam. Other interactions are likely to be reported as clinical experience with this drug increases. The clinical importance of these interactions is unclear.

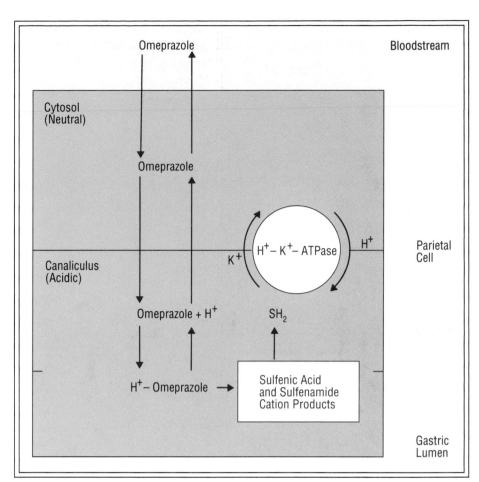

Figure 101A. Mechanism of omeprazole action.

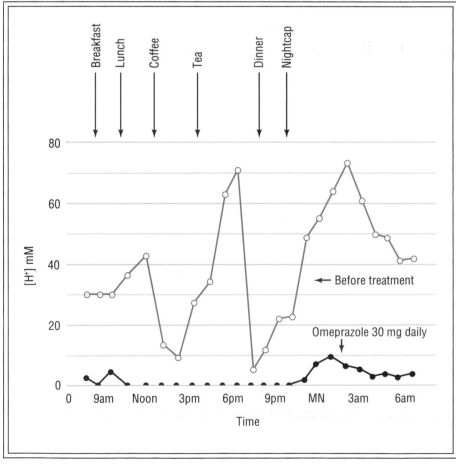

Figure 101B. Effect of omeprazole given at 9am on intragastric (H^+). Adapted from Walt et al, *Br Med J*, 1983;287:12-14.

Anticholinergic Therapy

Despite their effects on gastric acid secretion, there is only limited evidence supporting the efficacy of conventional anticholinergic agents in treating patients with peptic ulcer disease. Because anticholinergics may impede the outflow of gastric acid more than they reduce acid secretion in patients with peptic ulcer complicated by gastric retention, they are contraindicated in this clinical setting. These drugs are also contraindicated in patients with reflux esophagitis because they retard esophageal and gastric motility, reduce lower esophageal sphincter tone, and may actually enhance acid reflux. In addition, doses of these drugs that are sufficient to reduce secretion of gastric acid will also cause pupillary dilatation and a dry mouth and may precipitate urinary retention or an attack of glaucoma in susceptible individuals.

Because H_2-receptor antagonists block gastric acid secretion more effectively and have a more favorable safety profile, their introduction has largely supplanted the clinical use of conventional anticholinergic drugs in treating patients with peptic ulcer disease. Whereas atropine and other conventional anticholinergic drugs do not distinguish between the M_1 and M_2 subtypes of muscarinic cholinergic receptors, pirenzepine is a newly developed anticholinergic that is structurally similar to tricyclic antidepressant drugs (Figure 100). Pirenzepine binds tightly to M_1 muscarinic receptors on parietal cells, while binding only weakly to M_2 receptors on smooth muscle cells and exocrine glands. This selectivity results in an improved side-effect profile. Although pirenzepine is less potent than H_2 antagonists in inhibiting basal and stimulated secretion of gastric acid, it may be effective in providing pain relief and in promoting ulcer healing. It remains to be determined whether pirenzepine will have a role as initial therapy or as an adjunct to the use of H_2-receptor antagonists in treating patients with peptic ulcer disease.

Prostaglandins

Prostaglandins of the E and I series are normally synthesized by the gastric mucosa and function as endogenous inhibitors of acid secretion (Figure 94) and as cytoprotective agents (see below). Chemical modification of these compounds has resulted in a number of analogs that resist degradation after oral administration while retaining the ability to inhibit basal and stimulated secretion of gastric acid. Misoprostol is a synthetic prostaglandin (Figure 100) that has been shown to have therapeutic efficacy in patients with duodenal and gastric ulcers. Because misoprostol and other currently available analogs of prostaglandin E also stimulate intestinal secretion and motility, diarrhea occurs in a substantial number of patients and constitutes a major therapeutic drawback. These compounds cause uterine contractions and may induce abortions. For this reason these drugs are contraindicated in women who are pregnant or wish to become pregnant. Prostaglandin analogs are likely to remain second-line agents in the treatment of patients with peptic ulcer disease. They are particularly valuable as cytoprotective therapy in patients who require nonsteroidal anti-inflammatory agents.

Mucosal erosion and ulceration in acid-peptic diseases results from attachment and subsequent hydrolysis of mucosal proteins by pepsin. Acid facilitates this process by converting pepsinogen to pepsin, providing an acidic milieu that optimizes peptic activity (Figure 47), and by denaturing proteins, which increases their susceptibility to peptic hydrolysis. Both gastric and duodenal mucosa are covered with an adherent mucous layer, and the secretion of bicarbonate into this layer represents a primary cytoprotective defense against acid-peptic digestion (Figure 102). The gel formed by this bicarbonate-mucous layer retards the inward diffusion of H^+ ions. Because this gel is impermeable to large proteins (M.W. > 17,000), it effectively excludes pepsin (M.W. 35,000). There is an inverse relation between the rate of cell turnover and mucous secretion by gastric epithelial cells, and both epithelial cell life and mucous secretion are reduced in patients with gastric ulcers.

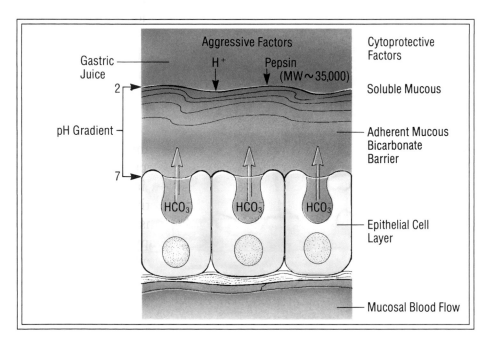

Figure 102. Aggressive and cytoprotective factors.

Secretion of bicarbonate is stimulated when the mucosa comes in contact with acid and other mild irritants but can be blocked by indomethacin and other inhibitors of cyclo-oxygenase, suggesting that this adaptive cytoprotection may be mediated to some extent by prostaglandins. This primary cytoprotective mechanism may be augmented by increasing mucosal blood flow or production of soluble mucous. Measures that neutralize or block the production of gastric acid also may have an important role in minimizing mucosal damage by peptic digestion. In theory, exogenously administered prostaglandins could enhance cytoprotection either by stimulating mucous and bicarbonate secretion or by increasing mucosal blood flow. Thus, it is often difficult to separate possible cytoprotective effects of these drugs from their effects on acid secretion.

In addition to prostaglandin analogs, two drugs have been developed that have primary cytoprotective actions and demonstrate the therapeutic utility of this approach.

Sucralfate

The observation that sulfated polysaccharides inhibit pepsin-mediated protein hydrolysis provided the impetus for developing a cytoprotective agent based on this principle. High molecular weight sulfated polysaccharides, such as heparin, have anticoagulant activity. However, antipeptic activity is related to the extent of sulfation rather than the molecular weight of the polysaccharide, and the octasulfate of sucrose was found to inhibit peptic hydrolysis *in vitro* and have antiulcer activity in experimental animals. When this compound was reacted with aluminum hydroxide, it formed a viscous, gel-like substance, called sucralfate, that is insoluble in water and has a weak buffering capacity.

Sucralfate is thought to function as a cytoprotective agent because negatively charged sulfate groups interact electrostatically with positively charged protein molecules, thereby preventing the formation of a complex between pepsin and these proteins that is a necessary first step before peptic hydrolysis (Figure 103). Because of its affinity for proteins and its viscosity and insolubility, sucralfate may form a physical coating over ulcer craters that retards the inward diffusion of acid and pepsin. The buffering capacity of sucralfate may augment the acid-neutralizing properties of the adherent mucous-bicarbonate layer and provide additional inactivation of pepsin. Sucralfate also binds bile salts that have been implicated in the pathogenesis of gastric ulcers.

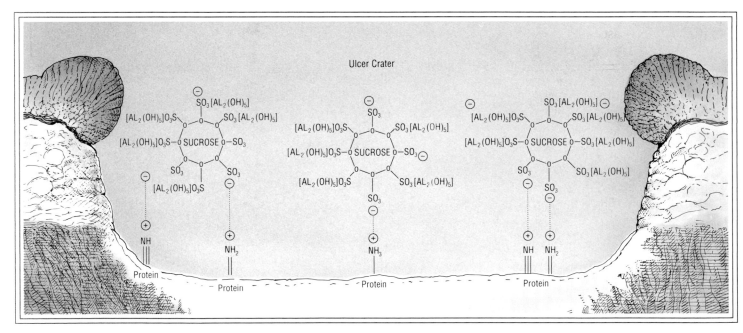

Figure 103. Sucralfate binds to tissue proteins in an ulcer crater.

Sucralfate has been shown to be effective in providing symptomatic relief and promoting healing of both gastric and duodenal ulcers. It is also effective in reducing ulcer recurrence. Side effects of sucralfate therapy have been limited to occasional constipation and symptoms of dry mouth. Sucralfate may also reduce the absorption of warfarin, digoxin, and phenytoin by about 20% when administered simultaneously with these agents. Because of its efficacy and safety, sucralfate can be used as a primary agent for the management of patients with peptic ulcer disease.

Colloidal bismuth subcitrate (CBS) is a complex bismuth salt of citric acid that at acid pH chelates with proteins in the ulcer base and may form a protective barrier against inward diffusion of acid and peptic digestion. This compound may also stimulate mucous secretion and has antibacterial activity against *Helicobacter pylori*, an organism that has been implicated in inflammation and recurrent ulceration of gastric and duodenal mucosa. CBS has been shown to be as effective as cimetidine in healing both gastric and duodenal ulcers and may also be efficacious in preventing ulcer recurrence. This latter fact has been cited to support the etiologic role of *H. pylori* in peptic ulcer disease because CBS has antibacterial activity not seen with H_2 antagonists. CBS uniformly causes patients to have black stools and, in some individuals, may cause darkening of the tongue, nausea, and diarrhea. Long-term therapy has been associated with an elevation in serum bismuth levels which may ultimately result in neurotoxicity.

In as much as reduced lower esophageal sphincter tone and gastric retention contribute to gastroesophageal reflux, cholinergic agents could ameliorate this condition by enhancing sphincter tone and increasing the rate of gastric emptying. Bethanechol, the first drug extensively evaluated for this purpose, reacts relatively selectively with muscarinic receptors on smooth muscle. It has a longer duration of action than acetylcholine because its carbamyl ester group resists hydrolysis by esterases (Figure 104). However, clinical experience with bethanechol has been generally disappointing, apparently because the drug does not significantly increase gastric emptying rate (Figure 105).

Colloidal Bismuth Subcitrate

Prokinetic Agents

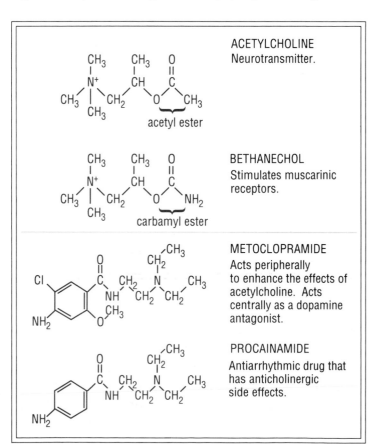

Figure 104. Prokinetic agents.

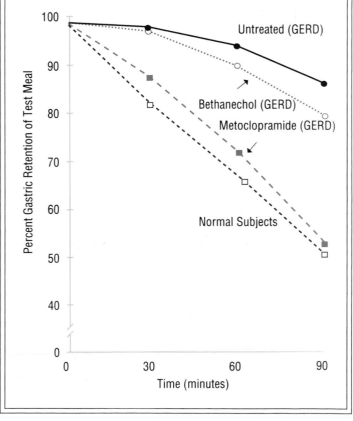

Figure 105. Acceleration of gastric emptying in patients with GERD by bethanechol and metoclopramide. Adapted from McCallum, et al, *Gastroenterology*, 1983;84:1573-1577.

On the other hand, metoclopramide not only increases lower esophageal sphincter tone but also the rate at which solid components of food are emptied from the stomach (Figure 105). Metoclopramide, a derivative of procainamide that bears no structural resemblance to conventional cholinergic compounds (Figure 104) has effects on gastrointestinal motility that can be blocked by atropine, but not by vagotomy. Thus, metoclopramide appears to act either by stimulating acetylcholine release from postganglionic cholinergic nerve terminals or by sensitizing muscarinic receptors on smooth muscle to acetylcholine. What distinguishes metoclopramide from bethanechol and other cholinergic agents is its ability to coordinate gastric, pyloric, and duodenal motor activity so that net aboral movement of gastric contents is optimized. For this reason, patients with reflux esophagitis accompanied by delayed gastric emptying may benefit when metoclopramide is used as an adjunct to therapy with antacids and H_2-receptor antagonists. Although definitive clinical trials are lacking, it is also possible that metoclopramide will benefit patients with gastric ulcer disease aggravated by duodeno-gastric reflux of bile.

Metoclopramide is also a dopamine antagonist, and this property may mediate some of its gastrointestinal effects as well as account for its frequently beneficial central anti-emetic actions. Inhibition of D_2 receptors in the anterior pituitary results in stimulation of prolactin release and, with long-term metoclopramide therapy, may lead to breast enlargement and galactorrhea. Drowsiness is the most common side effect of metoclopramide therapy. Extrapyramidal side effects, also mediated by central dopamine receptors, are less common but include akathisia and Parkinsonian and dystonic symptoms that primarily occur in children and patients with impaired renal function who receive excessive doses. As with other antagonists of dopamine receptors, the development of tardive dyskinesia has also been reported.

Plasma concentration-response relationships have not been established for the prokinetic effects of metoclopramide, but some central nervous system adverse effects are plasma concentration-dependent. Although a target plasma level of 1 ug/ml has been recommended when this drug is given intravenously to suppress nausea and vomiting in patients receiving cancer chemotherapy, levels of this magnitude will be poorly tolerated for prolonged periods since akathisia regularly occurs in patients on oral metoclopramide therapy when peak plasma concentrations exceed 120 ng/ml. Although the need for routine monitoring of plasma levels has not been established, plasma levels of metoclopramide have been used to demonstrate that the increased susceptibility of children to dystonic reactions has a pharmacodynamic rather than a pharmacokinetic basis. However, there appears to be a kinetic basis for adverse reactions in patients with impaired renal function, and the total elimination clearance of metoclopramide is reduced by 50% in functionally anephric patients. Since renal clearance accounts for only 25% to 40% of total metoclopramide clearance in normal subjects, both renal and nonrenal clearance of this drug must be reduced. Although strict application of the method shown in Figure 99 for individualizing drug dosage would be inappropriate, it can be anticipated that the dose of metoclopramide administered should be reduced by as much as half in patients with severely impaired renal function. Prokinetic agents thought to have a higher safety profile than metoclopramide include domperidone and cisapride.

An approach to managing patients with uncomplicated duodenal ulcer is schematized in Figure 106.

Approach to Patient Therapy
Duodenal Ulcer

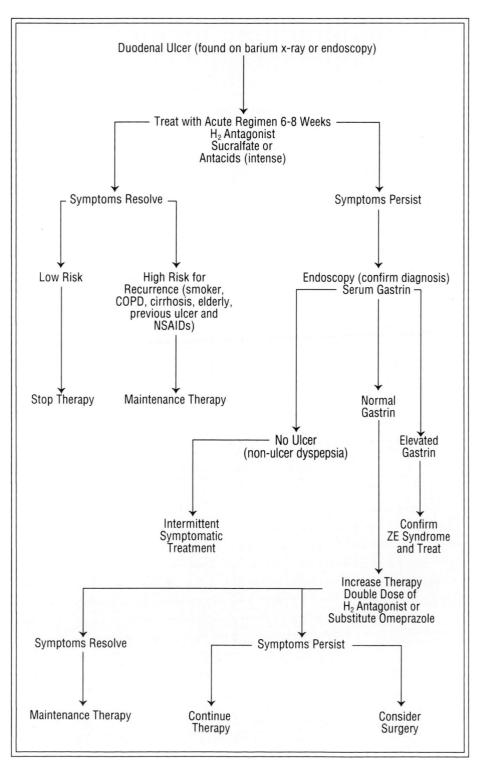

Figure 106. Management strategy for uncomplicated duodenal ulcer.

Pharmacotherapy should be combined with the general management principles that were outlined previously. Although antacids were the traditional mainstay of ulcer therapy, the introduction of newer drugs over the past two decades has provided more convenient therapeutic alternatives. Both H_2-receptor antagonists and sucralfate have been shown to lead to endoscopically verified ulcer healing rates of 60% to 75% within 4 weeks. Several therapeutic regimens that have approximately equal healing efficacy are summarized in Figure 107.

Figure 107. Equieffective oral therapeutic regimens for duodenal ulcer.

ANTACIDS	Maalox or Mylanta	30 ml 1 and 3 hours after meals and at bedtime
H_2-RECEPTOR ANTAGONISTS	Cimetidine	300 mg qid *or* 400 mg bid *or* 800 mg at bedtime
	Ranitidine	150 mg bid *or* 300 mg at bedtime
	Famotidine	20 mg bid *or* 40 mg at bedtime
	Nizatidine	150 mg bid *or* 300 mg at bedtime
CYTOPROTECTIVE AGENTS	Sucralfate	Before meals and at bedtime (stomach should be empty)

As experience with H_2-receptor antagonists has accumulated, it has been found that once-daily therapy aimed at reducing nocturnal secretion of acid has therapeutic effects that are comparable to the more frequent administration of several doses throughout the day. As previously emphasized, standard doses of H_2-receptor antagonists should be reduced appropriately in patients with impaired renal function. If antacids are used as ancillary agents, they should not be taken within 1 hour of an H_2-receptor antagonist or sucralfate.

When a duodenal ulcer is complicated by hemorrhage, penetration, perforation, or obstruction, hospitalization is necessary. A nasogastric tube should be placed initially for decompression and drainage of gastric contents and later for administering antacids and monitoring intragastric pH. Antacids or H_2-receptor antagonists should be given in a dosage sufficient to maintain intragastric pH above 4. This can usually be accomplished by administering at least 30 ml/hr of an aluminum and magnesium containing antacid preparation (Figure 91). Intravenous administration of H_2-receptor antagonists can also maintain intragastric pH above 5 when these agents are given by continuous infusion rather than by intermittent bolus injections (Figure 108). Because conventional doses of anti-ulcer agents have not been shown to affect the short-term course of patients with complicated duodenal ulcer disease, combination therapy with antacids and H_2-receptor antagonists has been used to raise intragastric pH to 7-8. pH changes of this magnitude not only inactivate but destroy pepsin and enhance hemostasis (Figure 109).

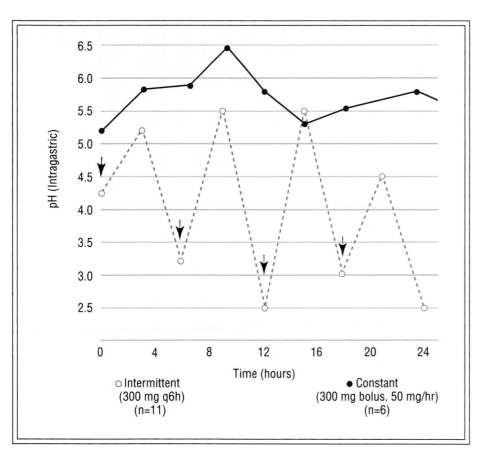

Figure 108. Comparison of intermittent (◆) and continuous infusion therapy with cimetidine. Adapted from Siepler, *Clin Ther,* 1986;8(Suppl. A):24-33.

Because omeprazole can also maintain achlorhydria for prolonged periods of time (Figure 101A), it may also be useful in this clinical setting. Intensive therapy with multiple agents may also be indicated for patients with intractable ulcers that are refractory to conventional management.

Recurrence is a prominent feature of the natural history of duodenal ulcers. More than three quarters of those patients who do not receive maintenance therapy can be expected to have recurrent symptomatic ulcers within 5 years after their initial episode. Accordingly, maintenance therapy is recommended for most patients. However, after 10 years, 95% become asymptomatic.

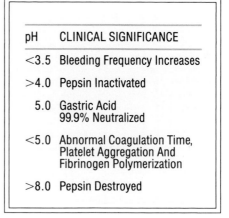

pH	CLINICAL SIGNIFICANCE
<3.5	Bleeding Frequency Increases
>4.0	Pepsin Inactivated
5.0	Gastric Acid 99.9% Neutralized
<5.0	Abnormal Coagulation Time, Platelet Aggregation And Fibrinogen Polymerization
>8.0	Pepsin Destroyed

Figure 109. Interpretation of intragastric pH values.

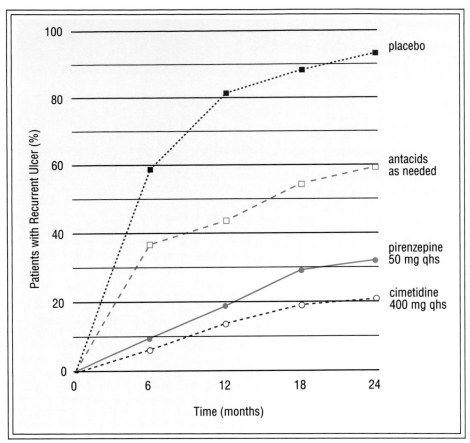

Figure 110. Recurrence rates for patients with healed duodenal ulcers. Adapted from Bresci et al, *Scand J Gastroenterol*, 1986;21(Suppl. 121):58-62.

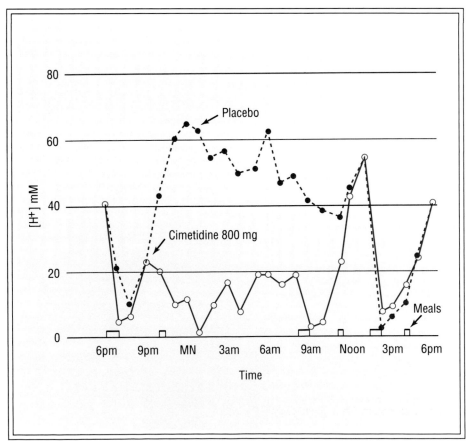

Figure 111. Reduction of intragastric (H^+) by cimetidine. Cimetidine or placebo was given at 8 pm. Adapted from Dammann et al, *Scand J Gastroenterol*, 1987;22(Suppl. 136):56-60.

Recurrence also increases the risk of complicating hemorrhage, perforation, and obstruction. For these reasons, patients whose ulcers recur after initial therapy should have a second full course of acute therapy and then be placed on an appropriate long-term maintenance regimen (Figure 110). Representative recurrence rates for patients treated with placebo, antacids as needed, pirenzepine, or cimetidine indicate that H_2-receptor antagonists are superior to antacids and anticholinergic agents (Figure 110). Evidence is mounting that reduction in nocturnal acid secretion is the most important factor in duodenal ulcer therapy and single bedtime dose regimens for cimetidine and other H_2-receptor antagonists not only effect substantial reductions in nocturnal acid secretion (Figure 111) but are also useful in maximizing patient compliance. There is limited evidence that twice daily administration of 1 gm sucralfate has equivalent efficacy in preventing recurrence in patients who cannot be maintained on H_2-receptor antagonists. In patients who relapse despite conventional maintenance therapy, it is reasonable to attempt long-term treatment with an acute healing regimen or with combined therapy with several anti-ulcer drugs or with omeprazole (Figure 106). Surgical intervention reliably alters the natural history of duodenal ulcer disease but is currently reserved for patients who do not respond to intensive pharmacologic measures.

An approach to managing patients with gastric ulcers is summarized in Figure 112. The frequency with which these ulcers occur in conjunction with gastric malignancy warrants the stringent use of endoscopy for biopsy and cytologic analysis. Surgery is indicated for patients who are found to be achlorhydric after pentagastrin stimulation. Once overt malignancy and achlorhydria have been excluded, treatment can be started with an acute healing regimen of an H_2-receptor antagonist or sucralfate as has been detailed for patients with duodenal ulcers. Recurrence is also common in patients with gastric ulcers, and maintenance dose regimens have been used to try to lower recurrence rates. Combined therapy with an H_2-receptor antagonist and sucralfate may provide benefits to patients who are resistant to either agent used alone.

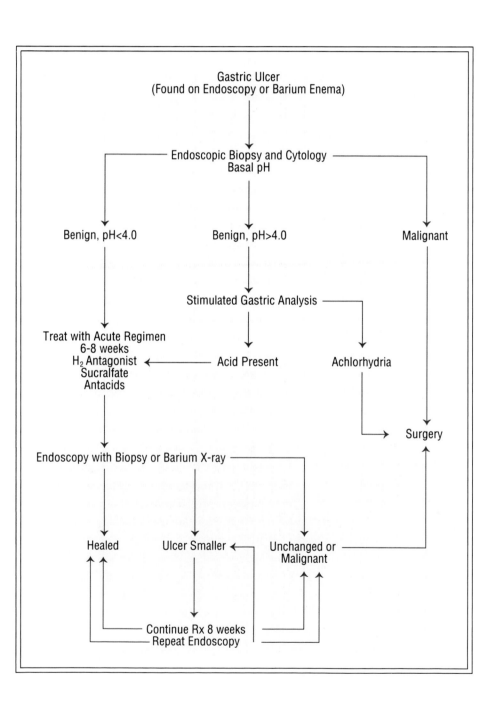

Figure 112. Management strategy for gastric ulcer.

Factors predisposing to stress ulceration are encountered in both medical and surgical patients and constitute an indication for prophylactic therapy (Figure 113). Stress ulcers are usually found in the acid producing areas of the gastric mucosa. They are characteristically superficial and seldom penetrate the muscularis mucosa. However, they are a major cause of severe gastrointestinal hemorrhage in critically ill patients. Curling's ulcers are acute gastric or duodenal ulcers developing in burn patients, whereas Cushing's ulcers are gastric or duodenal ulcers occurring in patients with central nervous system disease. Although clinically evident bleeding usually occurs 5 to 10 days after the precipitating event, superficial erosions may be found endoscopically within 24 hours. Therefore, aggressive prophylactic therapy is usually begun once patients at risk have been stabilized in an appropriate setting.

Antacids and H_2-receptor antagonists appear to have similar efficacy in preventing overt bleeding when used in the intensive regimens described above for patients with duodenal ulcers (Figure 114), and there may be some merit in using combined therapy to bring intragastric pH to 7 or above. Sucralfate, in a dose of 1 gm every 6 hours, also has been found to be an effective agent to prevent stress-related mucosal disease. Gastric colonization with gram negative bacteria is more extensive when gastric pH is elevated by antacids or H_2-receptor antagonists, whereas sucralfate has only minimal effects on gastric pH. Because gastric colonization has been correlated with retrograde bacterial spread to the pharynx and trachea, there is some concern that chronically intubated patients may have an increased rate of nosocomial pneumonia when gastric pH is elevated. Patients also may be at increased risk for developing nosocomial pneumonia if therapy involves increasing gastric volume.

TRAUMA/POSTOPERATIVE
Major Operative Procedure
Major Burns
Multiple Traumatic Injuries
Cranial Operations or Trauma
Hypovolemic Shock

MEDICAL
Respiratory Failure
Hepatic Failure with Jaundice
Renal Failure
Sepsis and Peritonitis

Figure 113. Indications for prophylaxis of stress ulcers.

Figure 114. Prevention of overt bleeding by cimetidine and antacids. Adapted from Shuman, et al, *Ann Intern Med*, 1987; 106:562-567.

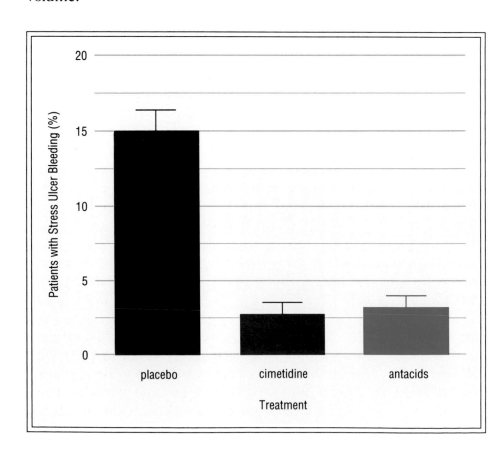

Although gastroesophageal reflux disease (GERD) has been estimated to produce daily symptoms, principally heartburn, in up to 10% of the U.S. population, most individuals treat themselves with over-the-counter antacid preparations and do not seek medical help. In fact, most patients with mild reflux esophagitis can be treated successfully with a program of lifestyle modifications and regular antacid therapy. These interventions are the cornerstone of the stepwise approach to managing patients with gastroesophageal reflux disease and have been designated as Phase I therapy (Figure 115).

Figure 115. Stepwise approach to therapy of gastroesophageal reflux disease.

PHASE I	Elevate head of bed at least 6" Stop smoking Eat a bland diet and avoid bedtime meals Avoid potentially harmful medications Institute regular therapy with antacids
PHASE IIA	Add therapy with H_2-receptor antagonists
PHASE IIB	Intensify therapy with H_2-receptor antagonists Add bethanechol or metoclopramide
PHASE IIC	Substitute omeprazole for H_2-receptor antagonist
PHASE III	Perform anti-reflux surgery

As a general principle, therapy for gastroesophageal reflux disease is designed to reduce gastric acidity, increase lower esophageal sphincter (LES) tone, and promote esophageal clearance of refluxed material. Elevating the head of the patient's bed has been shown to reduce esophageal exposure to acid. Smoking two cigarettes over a 20-minute period can reduce LES tone by as much as 50%, perhaps because inhaled nicotine blocks LES control mechanisms. Fatty foods, alcohol, and chocolates, which contain methyl xanthines, also impair LES function and should be avoided. Citrus juices, coffee, and spicy foods are direct irritants and may exacerbate symptoms. Since LES tone is reduced in the immediate postprandial period, patients should avoid lying down for several hours after eating. Theophylline (a methyl xanthine), classical anticholinergic agents, and progesterone delay gastric emptying and decrease LES tone; they are examples of medications that may exacerbate symptoms of gastroesophageal reflux. In fact, heartburn is a significant problem for many women during pregnancy. This is thought to be a consequence of physiologic increases in serum progesterone levels. Antacids have provided the initial approach to medical therapy and should be taken regularly 1 and 3 hours after meals and at bedtime.

Phase II therapy of gastroesophageal reflux disease includes a number of pharmacologic interventions designed to supplement Phase I management, but the general therapeutic principles are the same (Figure 116). An H_2-receptor antagonist should be added to the regimen of patients with mild-to-moderate symptoms that do not respond to 2 to 4 weeks of Phase I management and may be indicated as initial therapy of patients with more severe gastroesophageal disease (Phase IIA).

Figure 116. Phase II management of gastroesophageal reflux disease.

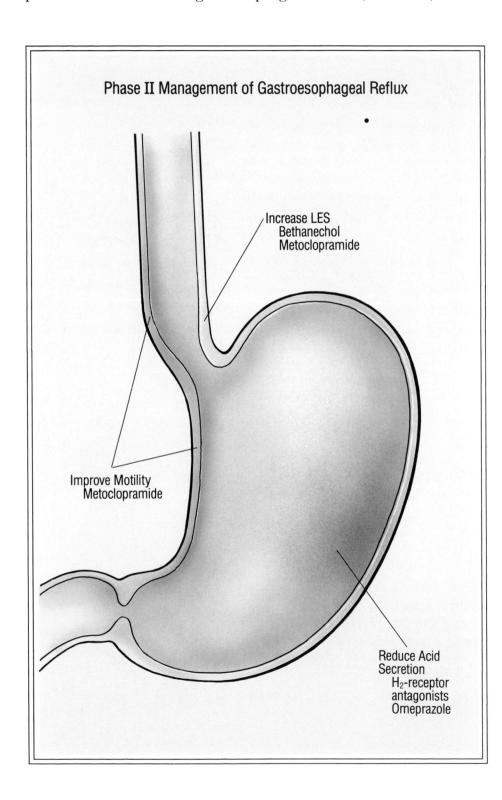

Symptomatic improvement may occur within a week of initiating therapy with an H_2-receptor antagonist. Treatment for 8 weeks is often required, however, to gauge the full extent of a therapeutic response

(Figure 117). If esophageal ulceration or erosion persist despite treatment with 3.2 g/day of cimetidine or the equivalent, patients may be considered as having refractory erosive esophagitis, and the measures designated as Phase IIB therapy are warranted. Bethanechol in a dose of 25 mg before meals and at bedtime may augment the efficacy of therapy with an H$_2$-receptor antagonist or omeprazole by increasing LES tone (Figure 116). Metoclopramide has similar effects on the LES and also may increase esophageal clearance and gastric emptying. The efficacy of metoclopramide is similar to that seen following administration of H$_2$-receptor antagonists (Figure 117). Therapy with metoclopramide is frequently associated with unacceptable neurologic or psychotropic adverse reactions, however, and this drug is best reserved for patients in whom delayed gastric emptying contributes to gastroesophageal reflux.

Omeprazole has been shown to have endoscopically verified healing rates that are superior to those observed with H$_2$-blockers (Figure 118) and only once-daily administration is required. Because experience with this drug is limited, it is currently reserved for patients in whom other medical therapy has failed (Phase IIC). Fewer than 10% of patients with gastroesophageal reflux disease will be refractory to medical management and thus require surgical intervention (Phase III). Even in responding patients, the natural course of gastroesophageal reflux disease is fluctuating, and the intensity of therapy should be varied accordingly (Figure 119).

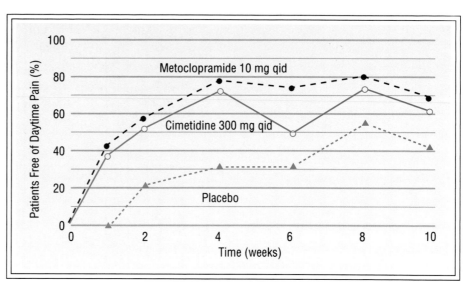

Figure 117. Relief of daytime heartburn pain with cimetidine and metoclopramide. Adapted from Bright-Asare, et al, *J Clin Gastroenterol*, 1980;2:149-156.

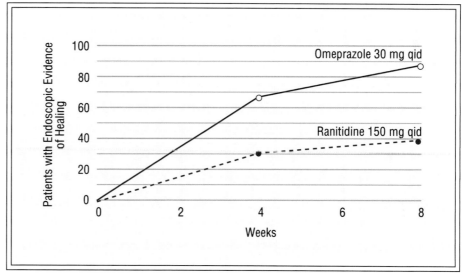

Figure 118. Comparison of GERD therapy with an H$_2$-receptor antagonist and a proton pump inhibitor. Adapted from Lundell, et al, *Gut*, 1987;28:A1375.

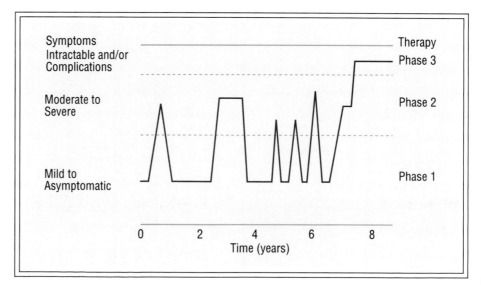

Figure 119. Timecourse of development of symptoms of GERD. Adapted from Richter, in *Gastro-esophageal Reflux Disease: Pathogenesis, Diagnosis, Therapy,* 1985.

General Therapeutic Considerations

Although general principles can be outlined for treating acid-peptic disease, successful clinical management requires integration of these principles in an individualized therapeutic regimen. This entails specific consideration of concurrent medical problems that may contraindicate certain therapeutic approaches, or may mandate reduced-dose therapy. For example, pregnant or possibly pregnant patients should not be treated with prostaglandins because of the abortifacient potential of these drugs. Because sucralfate is not absorbed, it may be preferred in pregnancy to drugs with systemic effects that have not been thoroughly evaluated in this clinical setting. However, the potential risk to the fetus from aluminum absorption which occurs in patients taking sucralfate or antacids containing aluminum hydroxide has not been examined.

Renal excretion of unmetabolized drug is the primary route of elimination of the available H_2-receptor antagonists (Figure 98) and of metoclopramide. Therefore, usual dose recommendations should be modified appropriately when these drugs are used to treat patients with impaired renal function. On the other hand, omeprazole is eliminated primarily by hepatic metabolism, and usual therapeutic doses are suitable even for functionally anephric patients. The dose of omeprazole may need to be reduced in patients with severe hepatic impairment.

Since patients are often treated concurrently with several drugs, potential drug interactions should also be considered. These drug interactions may be classified as either pharmacodynamic, when one drug interferes with the mechanism of action of a second drug, or pharmacokinetic, when one drug interferes with the absorption, distribution, or elimination of another. An example of a significant pharmacodynamic interaction is the reduction in gastric emptying rate caused by conventional anticholinergic drugs or drugs with anticholinergic side effects that may exacerbate symptoms of gastro-esophageal reflux disease. Representative pharmacokinetic interactions caused by drugs used to treat acid-peptic disease are summarized in Figure 120. The absorption-reducing effects of antacids and sucralfate can be minimized by providing a 1- to 2-hour interval between the administration of these agents and other therapies. Metoclopramide and anticholinergic drugs affect digoxin absorption because of their effects on small bowel

Interacting Drug	Affected Drug	Increased Absorption	Decreased Absorption	Decreased Metabolism	Decreased Renal Excretion
Antacids					
	Tetracycline		X		
	Digoxin		X		
	Cimetidine		X		
	Ranitidine		X		
	L-Dopa	X			
Cimetidine					
	Warfarin			X	
	Theophylline			X	
	Procainamide			X	X
	Phenytoin			X	
Ranitidine					
	Warfarin			X	
	Theophylline			X	
	Procainamide				X
Omeprazole					
	Phenytoin			X	
	Diazepam			X	
Sucralfate					
	Warfarin		X		
	Digoxin		X		
	Phenytoin		X		
Metoclopramide					
	Digoxin		X		
Anticholinergics					
	Digoxin	X			

Figure 120. Representative interactions caused by drugs used to treat acid-peptic disease.

motility. These interactions reflect the fact that the bioavailability of conventional tablet formulations of digoxin is such that the drug is not always well absorbed. This problem can be minimized by administering digoxin as an elixir or in liquid-filled capsules that have a faster dissolution rate. The interactions of cimetidine, ranitidine, and omeprazole with hepatic drug metabolizing enzymes have already been described. Cimetidine and ranitidine have been shown to impede renal tubular secretion of procainamide and its active metabolite. However, this effect is concentration-related and is less likely to be significant with ranitidine and other therapeutically more potent H_2-receptor antagonists.

Pharmacokinetic interactions do not constitute a contraindication to combined therapy with potentially interacting drugs. Such interactions should cause no additional inconvenience, for example, when theophylline is added to the regimen of a patient who has stabilized on cimetidine therapy. Individual variation in theophylline metabolism rates, even in patients not treated with cimetidine routinely, warrants using theophylline levels to guide dosing. On the other hand, if cimetidine or ranitidine is added to or withdrawn from the regimen of a patient who has been stabilized on theophylline therapy, additional theophylline dose adjustments should be anticipated, and theophylline levels should be monitored.

RECOMMENDED READING

1. Bertaccini G, Coruzzi G: Pharmacology of the treatment of peptic ulcer disease. *Dig Dis Sci* 1985;30:43S-51S.

2. Konturek SJ: Pharmacologic control of gastric acid secretion in peptic ulcer. *Mt Sinai J Med* 1983;50:457-467.

3. Halter F (ed): *Antacids in the Eighties*, Munich, Urban & Schwarzenberg, 1982, p 153.

4. Ganellin CR: A survey of recently described H_2-receptor histamine antagonists, in Gannelin CR, Schwartz JC (eds): *Frontiers in Histamine Research: A Tribute to Heinz Schild*, London, Pergamon, 1984, pp 47-59.

5. Clissold SP, Campoli-Richards M: Omeprazole: A preliminary review of its pharmacodynamic and pharmacokinetic properties and therapeutic potential in peptic ulcer disease and Zollinger-Ellison syndrome. *Drugs* 1986;32:15-47.

6. Albibi R, McCallum RW: Metoclopramide: Pharmacology and clinical application. *Ann Intern Med* 1983;98:86-95.

7. Porro GB, Petrillo M: The natural history of peptic ulcer disease: The influence of H_2-antagonist treatment. *Scand J Gastroenterol* 1986;21(suppl 121):46-52.

8. Strum WB: Prevention of duodenal ulcer recurrence. *Ann Intern Med* 1986;105:757-761.

9. Shuman RB, Schuster DP, Zuckerman GR: Prophylactic therapy for stress ulcer bleeding: A reappraisal. *Ann Intern Med* 1987;106:562-567.

10. Castell DO, Wu WC, Ott DJ (eds): *Gastro-esophageal Reflux Disease: Pathogenesis, Diagnosis, Therapy*. Mt Kisco, NY, Futura Publishing Co, Inc, 1985, p 324.

ACKNOWLEDGMENTS

Figure 24   Adapted from Nordgren B. The rate of secretion and electrolyte content of normal gastric juice. *Acta Physiol Scandinav,* 1963;58 (Suppl. 202):1-83.

Reprinted with permission from the publisher.

Figure 26   Adapted from Tang J. Evolution in the structure and function of carboxyl proteases. *Mole Cell Biochem,* 1979;26(2):93-109.

Reprinted with permission from the author.

Adapted from Andreeva NS, Gustchina AE. On the super-secondary structure of acid proteases. *Biochem Biophys Res Comm,* 1979;87(1):32-42.

Figure 27   Adapted from Donaldson RM. Intrinsic factor and the transport of cobalamin. In *Physiology of the Gastrointestinal Tract,* Second Edition, LR Johnson (ed), Raven Press, New York, 1987, p. 963.

Reprinted with permission from the author.

Figure 29   Adapted from Hinder RA, Kelly KA. Canine gastric emptying of solids and liquids. *Am J Physiol,* 1977;233(4):E335-E340.

Reprinted with permission from the author.

Adapted from Davenport HW. Salicylate damage to the gastric mucosal barrier. *N Engl J Med,* 1967;276:1312.

Reprinted with permission from the author.

Figure 40

Adapted from Wormsley KG, Grossman MI. Maximal histalog test in control subjects and patients with peptic ulcer. *Gut,* 1965;6:431.

Reprinted with permission from the author.

Figure 41

Adapted from Stremple JF, Molot MD, McNamara JJ, et al. Post-traumatic gastric bleeding. *Arch Surg,* 1972;105:179.

Reprinted with permission from the author.

Figure 42

Adapted from Pruitt BA, Foley FD, Moncrief JA. Curling's ulcer: A clinical-pathology study of 323 cases. *Ann Surg,* 1970;172:529.

Reprinted with permission from the author.

Figure 43

Adapted from Murray HS, Strottman MP, Cooke AR. Effect of several drugs on gastric potential difference in man. *Br Med J,* 1974;1:19-21.

Reprinted with permission from the author.

Figure 49

Adapted from Powell DW. Barrier function of epithelia. *Am J Physiol,* 1981;241:6275-6288.

Reprinted with permission from the author.

Figure 50

Adapted from Murthy SNS, Dinoso VP, Clearfield HR, et al. Simultaneous measurement of basal pancreatic, gastric acid secretion, plasma gastrin, and secretin during smoking. *Gastroenterology,* 1977;73:759.

Reprinted with permission from the author.

Figure 51

Adapted from Clamp JR, Allen A, Gibbons RA, et al. Structure of gastrointestinal mucus glycoproteins and the viscous and gel-forming properties of mucus. *Br Med Bull,* 1978;34:31.

Reprinted with permission from the publisher.

Figure 52

Adapted from Malagelada JR, Longstreth GF, Deering TB, et al. Gastric secretion and emptying after ordinary meals in duodenal ulcer. *Gastroenterology,* 1977;73:989-994.

Reprinted with permission from the author.

Figure 56

| Figure 57 | Adapted from Rotter JI, Sones JQ, Samloff IM, et al. Duodenal-ulcer disease associated with elevated serum pepsinogen I: An inherited autosomal dominant disorder. *N Engl J Med*, 1979;300:63-66.

Reprinted with permission from the author. |

| Figure 70 | Adapted from Fiddian-Green RG, McGough E, Pittenger G, et al. Predictive value of intramural pH and other risk factors for massive bleeding from stress ulceration. *Gastroenterology*, 1983;85:617.

Reprinted with permission from the author. |

| Figure 76 | Adapted from Demeester TR, Johnson LF, Joseph GJ, et al. Patterns of gastroesophageal reflux in health and disease. *Ann Surg*, 1976;184(4):463.

Reprinted with permission from the author. |

| Figure 89 | Adapted from Sontag S, Graham DY, Belsito A, et al. Cimetidine, smoking, and recurrence of duodenal ulcer. *N Engl J Med*, 1984;311:689-693.

Reprinted with permission from the author. |

| Figure 92 | Adapted from Milton-Thompson GJ. Monitoring of 24-hour acid secretion during antacid treatment. In *Antacids in the Eighties*, Halter F (ed), Urban & Schwarzberg, Munich, 1982, pp 72-79.

Reprinted with permission from the author. |

| Figure 101B | Adapted from Walt RE, Gomes Mde FA, Wood EC, et al. Effect of daily omeprazole on 24 hour intragastric acidity. *Br Med J*, 1983;287:12-14.

Reprinted with permission from the author. |

| Figure 105 | Adapted from McCallum RW, Fink SM, Lerner E, et al. Effects of metoclopramide and bethanechol on delayed gastric emptying present in gastroesophageal reflux patients. *Gastroenterology*, 1983;84:1573-1577.

Reprinted with permission from the author. |

| Figure 108 | Adapted from Siepler JK. A dosage alternative for H_2-receptor antagonists—constant infusion. *Clin Ther*, 1986;8 (Suppl. A):24-33.

Reprinted with permission from the author. |

Adapted from Bresci G, Capria A, Federici G, et al. Prevention of relapse with various antiulcer drugs. *Scand J Gastroenterol*, 1986;21 (Suppl. 121):58-62.   *Figure 110*

Reprinted with permission from the publisher.

Adapted from Dammann HG, Gottlieb WR, Walter TA, et al. The 24-hour acid suppression profile of nizatidine. *Scand J Gastroenterol*, 1987;22 (Suppl. 136):56-60.   *Figure 111*

Reprinted with permission from the author.

Adapted from Shuman RB, Schuster DP, Zuckerman GR. Prophylactic therapy for stress ulcer bleeding: A reappraisal. *Ann Intern Med*, 1987;106:562-567.   *Figure 114*

Reprinted with permission from the author.

Adapted from Bright-Asare P, El-Bassoussi M. Cimetidine metoclopramide, or placebo in the treatment of symptomatic gastroesophageal reflux. *J Clin Gastroenterol*, 1980;2:149-156.   *Figure 117*

Adapted from Lundell, et al. Omeprazole or ranitidine in the treatment of reflux esophagitis-result from a double blind, randomized, Scandinavian multi-centre study. *Gut*, 1987;28:A1375.   *Figure 118*

Adapted from Richter JE. Gastroesophageal reflux disease: A review of medical therapy. In *Gastroesophageal Reflux Disease: Pathogenesis, Diagnosis, Therapy*, Castell DO, Wu WC, Ott DJ (eds), Futura Publishing Co., Inc., Mt Kisco, NY, 1985, pp 221-241.   *Figure 119*

Reprinted with permission from the author.

Pathologic photographs provided by S.H. Saul, M.D.
Adjunct Associate Professor
Department of Pathology and Laboratory Medicine

Staff Pathologist
Chester County Hospital
West Chester, Pennsylvania

Radiographs provided by I. Laufer, M.D., Professor and Chief, Gastroenterology
Department of Medicine
University of Pennsylvania School of Medicine

PEPTIC ULCER DISEASE

Mechanisms & Management

EDITOR:

Perry B. Molinoff, M.D.
A.N. Richards Professor of Pharmacology
Chairman, Department of Pharmacology
University of Pennsylvania
School of Medicine
Philadelphia, Pennsylvania

CONTRIBUTING AUTHORS:

Arthur J. Atkinson, Jr., M.D.
Professor of Medicine and Pharmacology and Director of Clinical Pharmacology
Northwestern University Medical School, Chicago, Illinois

Jose Behar, M.D.
Professor of Medicine at Brown University and Associate Director, Division of
Gastroenterology at Rhode Island Hospital, Providence, Rhode Island

Robert M. Craig, M.D.
Associate Professor of Medicine and Chief, Gastroenterology
Northwestern University Medical School, Chicago, Illinois

James C. Reynolds, M.D.
Professor of Medicine and Chief, Division of Gastroenterology and Hepatology,
University of Pittsburgh, School of Medicine, Pittsburgh, Pennsylvania

MEDICAL ILLUSTRATOR:

Carol Donner, FAMI, SI
Santa Fe, New Mexico

The Healthpress Publishing Group, Inc.
Rutherford, New Jersey 07070